EXPLORING AND DEVELOPING THE USE OF ART-BASED GENOGRAMS IN FAMILY OF ORIGIN THERAPY

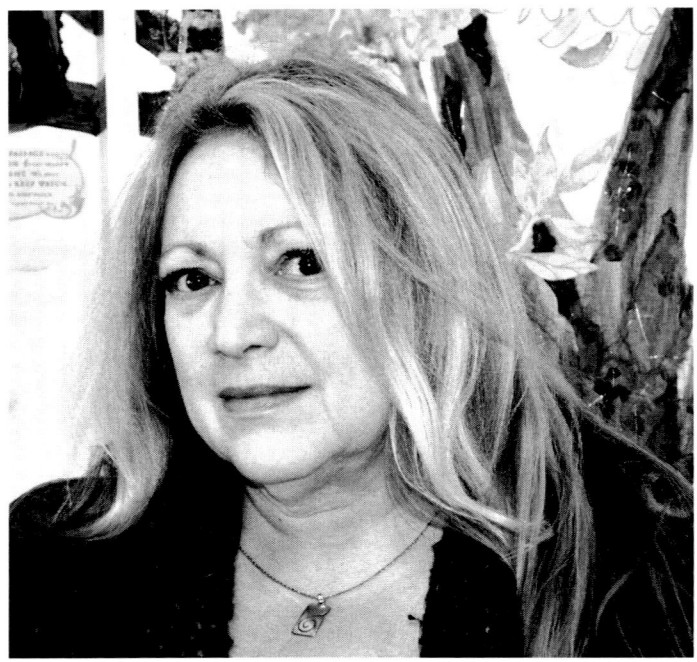

ABOUT THE AUTHOR

Deborah Schroder, ATR-BC, LPAT, is the chair of the Art Therapy/Counseling Program at Southwestern College in Santa Fe, New Mexico. She has intentionally worked with diverse populations in a wide range of settings. Her most recent clinical work has been with individuals and families, within a private practice, as time allows. A Midwesterner at heart, she graduated with an M.S. in art therapy and later taught at Mount Mary University in Milwaukee, Wisconsin, before moving to Santa Fe in 2002. She is an active member of the American Art Therapy Association. Her current professional commitment is encouraging and nurturing students as they take on the journey toward becoming art therapists. She likes to imagine the day when the professionals in the field of art therapy are as culturally and vibrantly diverse as the clients they serve. Passionate about exploring the international trends in art therapy, she has lectured and given workshops in Northern Ireland, Greece, Portugal, England and Italy. She is the author of *Little Windows into Art Therapy: Small Openings for Beginning Therapists.*

EXPLORING AND DEVELOPING THE USE OF ART-BASED GENOGRAMS IN FAMILY OF ORIGIN THERAPY

Sharing the Potential for Understanding and Healing Through the Art Process

By

DEBORAH SCHRODER, ATR-BC, LPAT

Chairperson, Art Therapy/Counseling Program
Southwestern College
Santa Fe, New Mexico

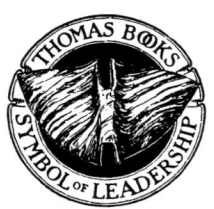

CHARLES C THOMAS • PUBLISHER, LTD.
Springfield • Illinois • U.S.A.

Published and Distributed Throughout the World by

CHARLES C THOMAS • PUBLISHER, LTD.
2600 South First Street
Springfield, Illinois 62704

This book is protected by copyright. No part of
it may be reproduced in any manner without written
permission from the publisher. All rights reserved

© 2015 by CHARLES C THOMAS • PUBLISHER, LTD.

ISBN 978-0-398-09071-5 (Paper)
ISBN 978-0-398-09072-2 (Ebook)

Library of Congress Catalog Card Number: 2015005644

With THOMAS BOOKS *careful attention is given to all details of manufacturing and design. It is the Publisher's desire to present books that are satisfactory as to their physical qualities and artistic possibilities and appropriate for their particular use.* THOMAS BOOKS *will be true to those laws of quality that assure a good name and good will.*

Printed in the United States of America
SM-R-3

Library of Congress Cataloging-in-Publication Data
Schroder, Deborah, 1957- , author.
 Exploring and developing the use of art-based genograms in family of origin therapy : sharing the potential for understanding and healing through the art process / by Deborah Schroder.
   p. ; cm.
 Includes bibliographical references and index.
 ISBN 978-0-398-09071-5 (pbk.) -- ISBN 978-0-398-09072-2 (ebook)
 I. Title.
 [DNLM: 1. Art Therapy. 2. Family Relations. 3. Pedigree. WM 450.5.A8]
 RC489.A7
 616.89'1656--dc23
                                                              2015005644

FOREWORD

This book embodies a genuine and personal look at the makeup of families and how previous individual family members affect future generations and carry forward past generational patterns. Art therapy provides a safe and respectful way to explore this information in a creative, uninhibited manner. The author shows the reader a new way of looking at recording these patterns by making the traditional genogram come alive through art therapy images. This process removes the art maker (student or client) from the limitations of square boxes and circles, allowing the true essence of each family member to burst through in metaphorical drawings and imagery.

The author takes this whole process one step further by acknowledging the importance and meaning of the art materials used, starting with the foundation on which the genogram is created. The foundation of the art-based genogram provides fruitful information about the family generational theme that is revealing and insightful for the art maker. It allows support for a creative depiction of the art maker's ancestral pain, sufferings, joys, celebrations and life viewpoints. Ultimately, this creative endeavor reveals therapeutic information that art makers can then integrate into their current, present-day lives.

As an art therapy graduate program director and professor, the author takes the reader step-by-step through the manner in which she teaches her students about art-based genograms in her Family Art Therapy classes. She does so by recounting various students' experiences with art-based genograms. Many of these stories reveal the internal and creative struggle students endure to come to an understanding of their families, and ultimately, to come to a resolution of past assumptions and beliefs. It is with compassion, respect and awe that the author provides a window into each story's unraveling and then reweaving of personal family perceptions. The core belief system of this art therapy program is that students must personally experience the art therapy intervention that they ask their future clients to do.

The author reveals her own vulnerability by displaying the results of her work in creating a personal art-based genogram and the cultural awareness ripple effect that resulted from her work on her family. She weaves personal acknowledgments of how her awareness of the world around her has become more attune with the historical patterns of the loved ones in her life. She discusses the intricacies of her daughter's adoption and how this affects her daughter's personal knowledge base and self-identity. The author discusses multicultural diversity, creating a unique view of how the art-based genogram influences the art makers' exploration of whom they are.

Throughout this book there is a fresh look at the power and effectiveness of art therapy. It demonstrates a wide variety of uses for art-based genograms in the teaching and professional preparation of art therapy graduate students, and ultimately, with art therapy clientele.

Deborah A. Good, Ph.D., ATR-BC, ATCS, LPAT, LPCC
Past President, The American Art Therapy Association
Past-President, The Art Therapy Credentials Board

PREFACE

I've been teaching Family Art Therapy for many years now. One of my requirements for this course is that each student create his or her own art-based genogram, and share it with the class. These art-based genograms are always visually fascinating and often emotionally challenging for the student to create.

Over and over we learn, in doing therapy, that it is imperative that we "do our own work." Requiring students to do their own work on who and where they come from is important to me. As we help our clients understand the gifts and struggles that they've taken on from their own family of origin, our ability to contain and hold the powerful emotions that come forward depends on our ability to stay centered and present as witnesses and guides.

This book was written after witnessing the power of using art in family of origin work with clients, and as part of my experience with my students. In my client work I can appreciate the urge that clients often have to "fix the problem." Sometimes we can explore the problem together without looking backwards. But often, we really need to understand the historical context for the patterns and beliefs that have influenced our lives. People make jokes about "blaming mom" when they talk about going to therapy. My interest in family history isn't ever to blame anyone. I'm much more excited about bringing our relatives' strengths and challenges and especially messages (conscious and unconscious) out into the open where choice is possible as one moves forward. And for me, the most meaningful and effective way to do that is through making art.

I would encourage anyone reading this book to create your own art-based genogram. I make a new one every time I teach my course and new insights, images and sometimes people, show up every year. I look at how I'm moving forward and what kind of emotional legacy I'm creating, and it all shows up rather magically in the messages within the art.

D.S.

INTRODUCTION

I remember the electric moment when I took those little squares and circles of my genogram and changed them out for images. It was magical! And I thought I was the first one to figure that magic out. Many other art therapists use shapes, lines, and color in genograms, and I'm proud to be one of the bunch, grateful as always to that large family of art therapists past, present, and future. Those first few sentences were all I wrote, originally, for this introduction. I was a little puzzled with myself – where had my other thoughts disappeared to? After some soul-searching, I found them.

Writing about generations of family inevitably resulted in my own deeply personal awareness of the assortment of roles that I've held over the years, including daughter, granddaughter, sister, partner, aunt, mother and grandmother. I touched into those fragile places at the intersections of good intentions and actual lived experiences, over and over again. I have some sadness associated with the word "family," and perhaps that somewhat accounts for my yearning to help people work on family of origin and generational family issues.

There is a sacredness to me in this talk about family. I hold tenderness around the hope that I carry, that family relationships can indeed "get better" and that all people have the right to show up, in family, in their own authenticity. The idea of choice is mentioned frequently in this book because it is critical. It is a treasure to choose what beliefs, rules, and ideas get taken in from all those generations before us. It is a treasure to expand who family can be and where we can connect in relationship. And the connections can be joyful. When one can touch joy in the midst of everything else that life brings, it feels miraculous.

ACKNOWLEDGMENTS

I want to thank my clients, colleagues, and students who have shared their art and stories with me. Client stories and art have been modified, and names and identifying details have been changed in order to protect confidentiality.

Leslie Monsalve-Jones, Larry Harkcom, and Claudia Escareno-Clark have such generous spirits and I appreciate their support and technical help. Claudia took many of the photos that appear in this book.

Dru Phoenix never wavered in her belief that this book should be written – her encouragement was priceless.

My heart has been touched by Wendy Wasserman's family stories and her perseverance to create an art-based genogram that she could be at peace with.

I was asking clients to create art-based family trees long before I really grasped the intricacies of Bowen's genograms. Art therapist Ruth Omlin gave me solid guidance in this area.

Heartfelt thanks to my partner Joey Esquipula Montoya, the solid, sheltering tree in my art-based genogram. And I'm so grateful for those two little bright spots of hope, my grandsons Elijah and Damian, who appear in my genogram as the adorable, cuddly little teddy bears that they truly are.

CONTENTS

	Page
Foreword	v
Preface	vii
Introduction	ix

Chapter

1. THE HISTORICAL USE OF GENOGRAMS 3
2. WHY ADD ART? 11
3. HOW TO CREATE ART-BASED GENOGRAMS 17
4. THE VALUE OF HISTORY IN A "HERE AND NOW" CONSCIOUSNESS 25
5. THERAPEUTIC USES IN INDIVIDUAL THERAPY 33
6. THERAPEUTIC USES IN COUPLES WORK 41
7. THERAPEUTIC USES IN FAMILY WORK 49
8. THE DOGGIE GENOGRAM, OR HOW TO WELCOME IN CHILDREN 55
9. GROUNDED IN THE DIRT 63
10. SAM'S STORY: RIDING A GLACIER 69
11. ALLIE CELEBRATES PEACH COBBLER 73
12. MULTICULTURAL GIFTS AND CHALLENGES REVEALED 77
13. THE INTERGENERATIONAL FLOW OF SPECIAL ISSUES 87

14.	TOXIC GREEN CHALK	95
15.	WIDENING OUR VIEWS, WORKING WITH COLLEAGUES	99
16.	RETURNING, FINDING MEANING	105

Epilogue 111
References 113
Index 117

ILLUSTRATIONS

Figure *Page*

1. Lillian's Family's Art-Based Genogram 4
2. Lillian's Family's Traditional Genogram 5
3. Oil Painting Genogram, Amy Hautman-Bates 19
4. Quilt Genogram, Candace Ayles 20
5. Chess Board Genogram, KaSandra Verett 21
6. Window Genogram, Kim Douglas 22
7. Teri's Genogram 64
8. Teri's Altered Book 66
9. Genogram Mobile, Sara Patrick 81
10. Tattoo, Val Jones 83
11. Dress, Laura Fischer 84
12. Rocks, Katherine Monroe 107
13. Game, Nancy Lemmon 110
14. Connecting the Dots, Wendy Wasserman 112

EXPLORING AND DEVELOPING THE USE OF ART-BASED GENOGRAMS IN FAMILY OF ORIGIN THERAPY

Chapter 1

THE HISTORICAL USE OF GENOGRAMS

There were two volcanoes in the image. One was huge, spewing hot orangey-red lava and deep black smoke, smeared across the paper with soft, messy chalk pastels. Molly and Tom had created the large volcano together, representing their father who was no longer living with them. Tom, who was fifteen, also created a smaller volcano as an image of himself. He had recently been involved in an intense physical fight at school, which was the reason that Lillian had brought her family to therapy. Thirteen-year-old Molly looked up with tears in her eyes. "Sometimes it's hard to be a turtle in this family – especially next to his volcano." She pointed to her brother's image. In the discussion that followed, there was no blame, just quiet talk of what they all used to do to try and prevent dad's temper from erupting. The red, oozing lava flowed toward each of them, encircling the turtle, and Molly (the turtle) was being ineffectively shielded by her mom, who had pictured herself as an umbrella. And Lillian, the umbrella, was exhausted (see Figure 1).

Painfully aware that she hadn't been able to shield her kids from her ex-husband's anger, she was terrified that Tom would turn into a huge volcano like his dad. Looking at the lava in the image we instinctively understood the overwhelming feeling of being surrounded by a family member's rage.

In future sessions we explored the effect of the raging lava on the turtle and the smaller volcano's lives, the relationship they formed and how their experiences of anger impacted all relationships in their lives. Tom felt like he had started out as a playful puppy and eventually he replaced his volcano in the art-based genogram with a jumping puppy. Lillian wondered if any of them would ever learn how to be angry in a healthy way.

Using the turtle image, Molly shared how she used to wonder every day if she would be the problem that would set off the tremors that would result in the volcano coming to life again. She talked about anxiety and insomnia and the urge to be invisible. She and her mom and brother had developed exquisite, finely-tuned antennae that they scanned their environments for danger with.

I share this particular case story because it captures the immediacy and accessibility of the images present in an art-based genogram. Emotions and relationship struggles were present, along with the gifts and strengths of family members. And in my enthusiasm I've jumped ahead of myself. It's important to understand the meaning behind genograms and they've been used.

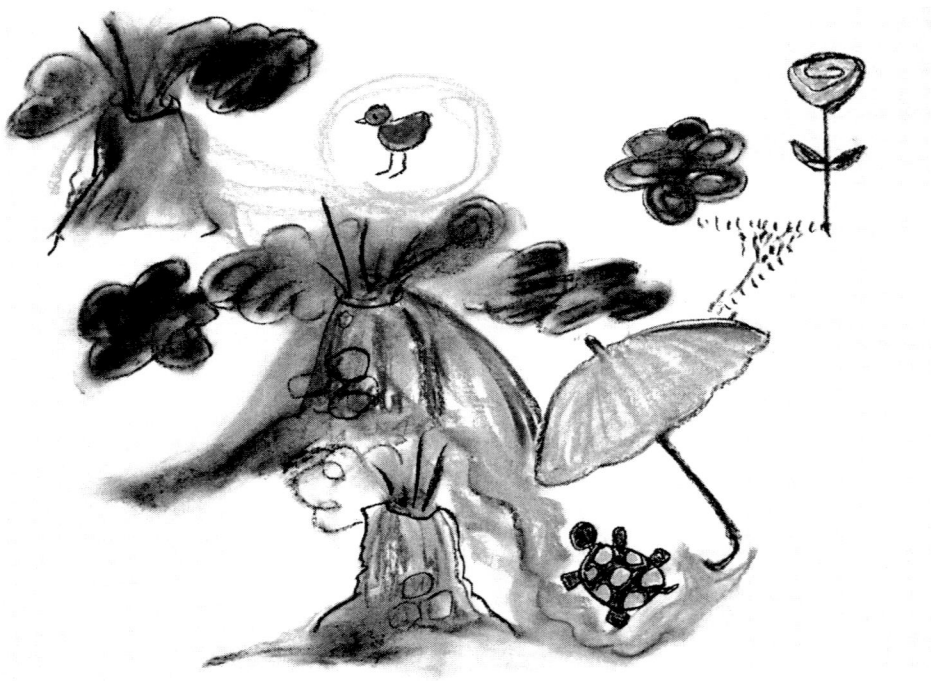

Figure 1. Lillian's Family's Art-Based Genogram.

The concept of the genogram didn't initially include art. Murray Bowen, well-known for his development of family systems theory, used

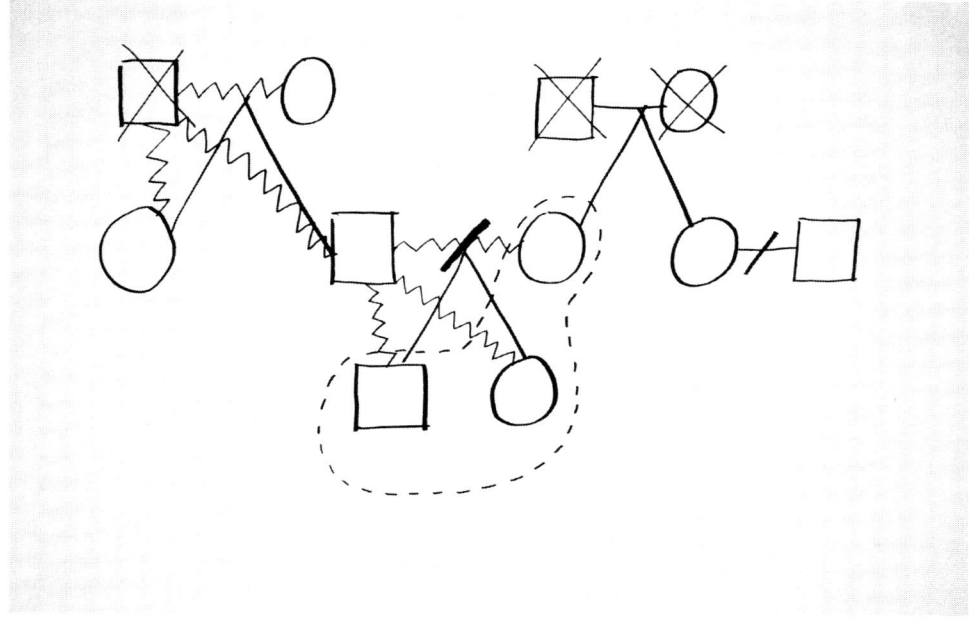

Figure 2. Lillian's Family's Traditional Genogram.

the concept of creating a sort of map of family members from the work of family physicians who tracked medical information generationally (McGoldrick, Gerson, & Petry, 2008). As Bowen mapped family members and important data including births, deaths, marriages, divorces, medical conditions, race, employment, etc. emerged, he developed ideas about how families intentionally and unintentionally transmit beliefs, emotional reactivity and ways of being family, across generations. He understood that his individual clients had been shaped and guided by many generations of their ancestors, either consciously or unconsciously. Bowen stated: "After having spent thousands of hours sitting with families, it became increasingly impossible to see a single-person without 'seeing' his total family sitting like phantoms alongside him" (Bowen, 1978, p. 152).

On the first day of my family art therapy course I always invite my students to understand that the room will be filled, every class, with our ancestors. As we start sorting them all out, I think it's important to first understand and use the traditional genogram and I encourage them to explore McGoldrick's thorough examples (McGoldrick, Gerson, & Petry, 2008). I also like to show clients the traditional structure as a beginning, organizational exercise (see Figure 2). The value of having a structure to create a family map with always becomes apparent quickly. "Genograms allow you to map the family structure clearly and to note and update the map of family patterns of relationships and functioning as they emerge" (McGoldrick, Gerson, & Petry, 2008, p. 3).

People often discover gaps in what they know about their families. While many families have a sort of "family historian," some families haven't written names and connections down. I often hear clients say things like "I don't know much about that side of the family. Nobody ever talked about them." It can be useful homework for people to do a little digging and make some inquiries. "The process of collecting information using a genogram is therapeutic in itself. Often the conversation about repetition of family patterns, significant events, and concurrent life stresses that occurs while doing the genogram will encourage a dialogue that helps families to see multiple possibilities and outcomes" (McGoldrick, Gerson, & Petry, 2008, p. 253). Family research and the creation of the genogram reveal "magical aspects of the family that have been hidden from family members – secrets of their history. Such revelations help families understand their current dilemmas and provide future solutions" (2008, p. 9).

In a discussion of beliefs about family, Virginia Satir listed these six beliefs that she held:

> *Every family member has to have a place.* Simply because he is a human being and is present. . . . *Every family member is related to every other family member.* . . . *Every family member is potentially the focus of many pulls* simply because he has so many relationships. . . . *Since the family develops over time,* it is always building on what it has already developed. . . . *Every family member wears at least three role-hats* with which he lives and through which he lives. (1972, p. 169)

It's that fourth belief that seems important to elaborate on here – the idea that as the family develops, it's building on its own past: "We always stand on what has been built before. Therefore, to understand what is going on in the present, one needs a perspective of the past. I would add that a past seen in terms of experience and the resultant learning therefrom will usually illuminate the present, and never mind about labeling it right or wrong" (1972, p. 169).

When we have enough basic family information to complete an initial family map, we can move on to the art making which will move the genogram into a deeper place, a place informed by psyche or soul — that place where our creative, intuitive voices whisper. An art-based genogram will allow the intuitive whispers to become heard and their images made visible.

I honestly don't know what Bowen would have thought about creating genograms filled with art and imagery. My belief is that the unconscious, where family beliefs, rules, traumas and strengths exist, can be seen and heard primarily through engaging one's creative process, which bypasses the editing, filtering and rules against sharing information that may be one's conscious, lived experience.

Through examining genograms Bowen could track two important variables in generations of family life, differentiation and togetherness.

> Family systems theory assumes the existence of an instinctually rooted life force (differentiation or individuality) in every human being that propels the developing child to grow to be an emotionally separate person, an individual with the ability to think, feel, and act for himself. Also assumed is the existence of an instinctually rooted life force (togetherness) that propels child and family to remain emotionally connected and to operate in reaction to one another. (Kerr & Bowen, 1988, p. 95)

I am reminded of the great lengths that young adults often go to in order to proclaim themselves as independent beings who are not anything like their parents or relatives. This is a normal developmental process, and while adult relatives may joke about it, applaud it, or secretly fear it, there aren't many acknowledged methods for moving through it with any grace. Many cultures have beautiful coming-of-age rituals, and unfortunately many United States families have no cultural reference point for this important tradition. It also is important to note that the idea of family togetherness and connection to a larger cultural community creates many different ideas of what being a part of a family should look like. There are, happily, many versions of what the togetherness force can look like in the context of a community; an idea that will be further addressed in Chapter 12.

Young adults of all cultural backgrounds often try the "geographical cure" and move across the country or out of the country altogether in order to claim some degree of individuation. Most discover that the move won't magically bestow a happy, healthy adulthood upon them. And so the dilemma of how to be one's own individual self while also maintaining family attachment, continues on.

> In broad terms, the togetherness force defines family members as being alike in terms of important beliefs, philosophies, life principles, and feelings . . . the differentiating force places the same kind of emphasis on 'I'. . . . This is the responsible 'I', which also assumes responsibility for one's own happiness and comfort and well-being. (Bowen, 1978, p. 218)

My young client Tom was clearly struggling with what kind of grown-up male he would become. It would be easy to become another volcano in a family history loaded with explosive relatives. His own development was much more complicated than choosing to be a happy dog who had learned some anger management, in the art-based genogram. He and his sister and mom were interested in the harder, more complicated work of defining what family beliefs, strengths and gifts could be built upon or developed, and what would be discarded, while allowing each family member to show up in life as their own authentic selves. I believe that I was able to challenge them to treasure both the authenticity of each individual and their connection as family, through the honesty and power of the art. The honesty of the art can be a little unsettling. Sometimes I feel like the art is a mischievous pixie, surprising my clients with weighty, existential truths when they least expect it.

My client Faith had moved back to New Mexico to help care for her mother who was undergoing treatment for cancer. Her father had died a few years before. Faith was a teacher and found work easily enough, but wasn't crazy about moving back to the desert from the northwest. She was interested in doing some "quick work" in order to "stop snapping" at family members.

And it was a big family. I felt a little confused when Faith spoke about who was who, and what the connections were like. It felt vital to me that we map this big group out and so I shared the idea of the genogram with her. She used different colors to fill in the traditional squares and circles, and the colors indicated a variety of medical and emotional issues. I could tell that she was getting frustrated with me when I was curious about some of the issues that were showing up. There was a lot of red flowing through her genogram, which was her color for heart disease. The only orange circle, her color for cancer, was her mother.

I think that I said something like "I see your mother is the only one that's colored orange," and I was surprised by her angry response: "Shit happens. That's all there is to it." She picked up a dark brown crayon and colored in one of the circles representing a sister. She was coloring with force and I watched quietly. "This is Eva. She took our mother to someone who supposedly did something to mom's aura or chakras." Then she pointed to another circle/sister: "This is Ruthie who takes mom to an herbalist, an energy-healer, whatever that is, and weekly acupuncture."

We sat silently and then I gently touched the orange circle and said "It sounds like your mother is well-loved." Faith looked teary and her face became red. "I take her to the real doctors. I pick up her prescriptions. I put the pills in the little boxes for daily doses. I'm the only one who takes this seriously!"

As I got to know Faith I heard the story of someone who had left home as soon as she could. She described her upbringing as "anything goes," in a family that meditated, grew their own organic vegetables and sought alternative health providers long before any of that was considered more mainstream. Faith shared: "My friends called us granolas. My clothes were sewn at home or bought at thrift stores. I couldn't wait to get out. I used to try and convince my brothers and sisters that there is a big, different world out there, but I'm the only one who moved away."

There's a story, based on Plato's myth of the cave, that speaks to the loneliness of being the only fish in a small pond who has seen glimpses of the larger world. The fish named Small Fry was scooped up by the Great Bird of the Mountain and given a sightseeing tour of the World Beyond the Pond (Kronberg & McKissack, 1990). Coming back to the pond was difficult, to say the least. I shared the story with Faith and invited her to draw a circle around everyone in the genogram who was "in the pond." Then I asked her to put some images about life in the pond, inside the circle, and images that represented the bigger world, outside the circled area. This art process took place over several sessions and as it moved forward, the tendency toward black and white thinking shifted enough that there were "good" and "bad" things inside and outside the pond of home.

The deep fear that emerged from her genogram was centered around Faith's own mortality as she contemplated the idea that her mother might die. There was almost a quality of panic surrounding the fear that Faith, too, might die back here, even though she had successfully left long ago. She was back and metaphorically swimming frantically.

Her genogram had given her a map of the family pond. I like to think that if she did make it out into the larger world again, that perhaps she had a clearer sense of herself as a member of her family and an appreciation for the positive family qualities that she carried within her.

Chapter 2

WHY ADD ART?

When I first encountered the traditional genogram and read about its uses, I remember being struck by the inherent visual appeal. Here was a map of the family! Something to look at that told a story. As an art therapist I immediately wondered what might happen if I switched out the squares and circles for color and image. So I tried it, experimenting first with my own family genogram.

I began by creating the standard genogram so that I had a map to follow. I experimented with the crossed-out square that represented one of my grandfathers. In traditional genograms, an "x" across a circle or square indicates death, and birth and death dates are often added in. But my purpose was not to record his death but to bring my memories of him and our relationship, to life. First I drew a little factory, remembering his hard work building tractors. But then I thought about a more personal image. I doubt if he loved the factory, but he did love his garden. Every inch of it was carefully tended with no wasted space. Lush vegetable plants along with the brilliant colors of his gladiolas filled every possible little plot in their small backyard. He placed tiny "treasures" like pretty marbles in the garden that enchanted me when I "helped" him. So his symbol on the genogram became a little garden patch. I soon realized that an art-based genogram required larger paper!

Next I created a symbol for grandma. A bowl of chocolate pudding seemed perfect since she always made that special treat for me when I spent the night. The beginning of my lifelong relationship with chocolate.

People and memories were coming to life! Soon each grandparent had his or her own symbol and there was no "crossing out" people who had died because they each remain present to me, not only in my memories but perhaps more importantly, in my own understanding of who I am as a person.

My siblings and my own children became colorful and present in a much more vibrant way, on the page. I noticed similar colors and images used for my youngest sister and my youngest son. What shared traits were apparent and how was my relationship with each of them reflected in the symbols that I chose for them both? By turning the genogram squares and circles into pictures I had opened up some new things to think about in my relationships.

Both my youngest sister and my youngest son had symbols that reflected their happy spirits and good-natured optimism. A yellow smiling sun represented my sister and a yellow cup of coffee symbolized my son. At the time he worked at a coffee shop but I chose the coffee cup because when he came to visit we would sit for hours over coffee, catching up with one another. A warm memory surfaced when I looked at the buttery color of the coffee cup – his "blankie" had been yellow.

Another sweet similarity surfaced when I sat with my completed art-based genogram. I used roses to represent both my daughter Grace and my grandma Martha. On the surface these two women wouldn't appear to have much in common. In my image, grandma Martha is a pink rose which for me, speaks to her kind, gentle presence in my childhood. Grace is a deep red rose in the image, strong and present in life with independence and persistence. As she has grown as a young mother, though, I've enjoyed seeing a tender gentleness appear and flourish within her and so I unconsciously visually linked her to my grandmother. Art welcomes these unconscious understandings out into the open, making them visible and conscious.

As the lines of the traditional genogram gave way to more art-based lines, bolder statements of meaning became clear. Jagged lines between squares and circles can suggest difficult relationships, but the jagged line can't speak to the emotional, felt experience or meaning of a difficult relationship. But a fish swimming away from a small pink kitten tells a deeper story. There is a cold indifference, a willingness to disconnect, in the fish's wake. A sadness is evident in the kitten's isolation. A perfect example of two people marrying young, terribly undifferentiated, according to Bowen's model. If each could have been their authentic adult selves it would have been clear that kittens and fish aren't compatible. Instead, many years went by as the fish swam away through golf, hunting, and ironically, fishing.

Convinced of the power of imagery I began asking my clients to let their family members show up as symbols or pictures in genograms. I was reminded of one of art therapy's founders and the family art therapy evaluation that she created. Hanna Yaxa Kwiatkowska was well known as an artist before she entered the field of art therapy during its beginning years as a profession, studying with Margaret Naumberg (considered one of the mothers of the field in the United States). Kwiatkowska worked for the National Institute of Mental Health and became a pioneer in the use of art therapy with families (Kwiatkowska, 1978).

She created a sequence of art tasks that she asked family members to complete. The third task was an abstract family portrait. She spoke of what happens when the family members are finished with their drawings: ". . . spontaneous discussion usually ensues because each person wants to know the meaning of a particular symbol by which he is represented" (Kwiatkowska, 1978, p. 88). She considered the abstract family portraits to be "the most interesting of all the procedures: they bring up many highly charged feelings and are the climactic point of the session" (Kwiatkowska, 1978, p. 88). This seems to me to be therapeutic movement allowing family members to begin experimenting with sharing authentic feelings with one another. That principle becomes amplified in the art-based genogram.

Choosing symbols to represent family members is often a good therapeutic challenge. It can be difficult for clients as it requires them to move into their feelings and memories – something that drawing a square or circle doesn't necessarily require. If done in individual therapy, my client may really struggle to identify the "correct" symbol. I encourage clients, though, to use their intuition and first impulse and I invite people to create more than one symbol for a family member, if needed. The difficulty of the process simply speaks to the complicated memories and relationships with family members.

One of my clients, Nan, needed to take a separate paper and create the contrasting images that came to mind when she thought about her aunt who she had lived with during her high school years. First she took chalk pastels and created a swirl of pink clouds. She remembered, as a little girl, feeling surrounded by softness and warmth when her aunt came to visit. Years later, after Nan attempted to run away from home, she was sent to live with her aunt. Now her memories shifted and Nan took crayons and drew a little house with black and white walls and roof; everything had seemed "black and white, good or bad" during those years with her aunt.

When Nan thought about her current relationship with her aunt, it seemed to her that there was much emotional distance now that Nan was an adult. She decided to draw a little bird perched on the top of a black and white birdhouse. The image didn't seem complete to Nan until she smeared a little pink cloud around the birdhouse.

A similar struggle may happen when a family creates a genogram together. I ask the family members to work on the same large paper and talk about how they will portray themselves and their extended family. People may have trouble, for example, determining a single symbol for grandpa. Perhaps dad remembers him as stern and wants to represent him as a guard dog. But mom experienced him as solid, perhaps a rock, and little daughter sees him as a teddy bear.

The discussion of family members' perceptions is extremely helpful for understanding the myriad relationships and roles a person can hold in family life. So instead of a square depicting grandpa, we have a guard dog, a rock and a teddy bear, clustered together – a much richer representation in terms of visual, and most importantly, emotional information.

In my own family, one of my sisters had different memories of my "chocolate pudding" grandma. Mary and I are eight years apart and of course had different relationships with each grandparent. She remembers grandma telling scary bedtime stories. I'm not sure what she'd create for grandma on an art-based genogram!

Sometimes the background of the image is important to represent. The geographic location of the family may speak volumes about the cultural beliefs in forming the client's history. Clients may need to draw or paint in the landscape of where the family came from. One genogram contained the lush green of Ireland, the cornfields of Iowa and the ocean and beaches of California where one branch of the family had settled.

As memories and family strengths and challenges were shared through the art, it became clear that family rules and beliefs had been passed down from Irish relatives. Within the branch of the family that settled in Iowa, those beliefs had taken on a midwestern flavor, as the family gained land and became settled in a small town. The branch that settled in California seemed to have changed the most in terms of the qualities valued in family life. It is important to note that the genogram was created by a part of the family who had lived in California and then moved to New Mexico. It was their perception that the Iowa side of the family held more tightly to tradition and ways of being family. Part of their discussion centered on what family values they would like to rediscover and which changes made historically in California, had been useful to them.

One family member had recently visited with some of the Iowa relatives while on a business trip to Des Moines. She had thoroughly enjoyed having dinner with her distant cousins and her visit had included going along to watch a softball game that the fourteen-year-old was playing in. When Shelly returned to New Mexico she shared with her spouse and kids that their Iowa relatives made a point to spend most dinners together. Although this idea was met with some eye-rolling, Shelly and her family agreed that dinner three times a week would help them all feel more connected.

A shift in religious practice had happened with the branch of the California family and the newly transplanted Californians weren't clear about the importance of that part of life. In California the family had gradually dropped Catholicism, and tended to describe themselves as spiritual but not attached to a faith community. It was interesting that once settled in New Mexico, Shelly's husband became interested in and moved by the rituals of the Catholic Church which is such a strong influence in the lives of many New Mexicans.

Another client created a beautiful backdrop for her genogram that included desert and mountains on the left side of the paper and a beach with waves lapping at the shore, on the right. The image that she chose to represent herself with was an elk. Her family members were painted as a variety of sea creatures. She had never felt like she "fit in" with her family and had moved across the country from Georgia to New Mexico. The geographic leap had certainly quieted some of the friction that she'd experienced with her family but as often is the case, the move didn't serve the individuation process in the manner that she hoped it would.

Sitting with her genogram and seeing her relatives as sea creatures and herself as an elk, led to some important realizations about how hard it was to love and miss her sea creature family. We used the metaphors to explore the sorrow of an elk who can't share who she is with a jellyfish. They can't even tolerate the same environments – how will they attempt to communicate? They hold very different principles and values as dear to their hearts, and my client was able to talk about the sadness that she carried with her about never feeling understood by her family. And there was a little creative whimsy present as she fantasized about being an elk that came from three generations of sea creatures, and what kind of possibilities the future for this family might hold. Image-making allows us to play with different endings to a story.

My clients have tended to use fairly traditional drawing and painting materials when creating their art-based genograms. The elk and her sea creature relatives were drawn with markers and filled in with watercolor paint. It has been in my students' art-based genograms that I saw the variations in media choice become excitingly clear.

Chapter 3

HOW TO CREATE ART-BASED GENOGRAMS

I suspect that my graduate students get tired of me talking about getting-to-know-you art. During supervision, student therapists sometimes talk about becoming swept up in what can seem like constant talking by a new client. I have much compassion for that situation because I think it's normal for people to wait to come to therapy until they're literally ready to explode from the need to be seen and heard. Helping someone feel seen and heard is an enormous privilege in this work, and we all know that being swept away by a wild flowing river of talk, week after week, probably won't be helpful in the development of a solid therapeutic relationship. So if I can help my students learn how to divert that river into a quiet art-making lake, they'll have the opportunity to welcome stillness, quiet, peace, into the room and have the opportunity to get to know the client in a deeper way.

I consider this getting-to-know-you art precious to the development of a therapeutic relationship, and I think that encouraging a person to "show up" visually, whether it is a collage of magazine pictures or a splash of watercolor that shares this moment's feeling, moves a person to a fuller metaphysical vocabulary. And so the beginning of an art-based genogram can simply be an image or symbol of oneself. And we need to communicate to our clients the wider spaciousness of that request without creating a bigness that can't be grounded in an image. So, simple words, few words, have worked well for me. "Let's start with an image that would share with me something about you today."

An image grounded in today frees someone from trying to identify some kind of ultimate self-symbol that incorporates all aspects of one's being and multiplicity of roles. In other words, my initial response to creating an image representing me, right now, doesn't have to include me as mom, me as friend, me as art therapist and me ten years ago.

I trust the client to move toward the art materials that seem appealing. A client's art vocabulary may grow in our work together and while I applaud risk-taking with different media choices, the art material chosen doesn't determine the value of the self-image that appears. A client took a piece of black yarn and tied knot after knot in it, twisting and tying it into a complicated tangle of yarn about two inches in diameter. That became the beginning of her genogram. We spent time sitting with the little tangle of yarn and she cried when she explained why this was who she was that day.

Her next step was to envision her parents, using art, and their images were different insects created with markers. It took three sessions to work with the black tangled yarn and the two insects. She cut out the insect pictures and moved them around, trying out different visual distances between them all. It was important to Leanne to start by sharing stories, sharing memories that had shaped her sense of distance and placement with the genogram.

Other people prefer to start from a more traditional, organizational place, perhaps using the language of squares and circles to map out "who goes where" before shifting into art. Southwestern College student Amy began with the traditional format but quickly became frustrated. In her piece for the Southwestern College blog, titled *Mapping Out Family Systems with Genogram Oil Painting,* Amy spoke about her genogram experience saying that she absolutely couldn't deal with trying to fit her family into any kind of box or system. She found success, though:

> Then, while hiking one day, I came upon a ridge topped with jagged dark iron rich boulders carved with ancient petroglyphs. Primitive symbols of humans, birds, spirals and crosses were etched in the sun facing surfaces . . . thinking about the history of the place, I looked out over the hills and wondered how many people had stood in this very spot, contemplating life. . . .
>
> These marks of history, carved in stone, were the inspiration for my genogram (see Figure 3). I started with an ochre base and then laid a dark patina over the entire canvas. I wiped off a circle of burnt umber to reveal myself as a golden sun shedding light on the family system I know. Then, scratching into the surface, figures began to emerge. In the shadows of the upper left is my grandpa Smed, a colorful character who died of cirrhosis.

But I wanted to show more than a dead alcoholic patriarch. So I gave him a jester quality to convey his humor and importance.

At the bottom of the canvas are my two children. They are portrayed as neutral and whole. I didn't want to smear them with red, or aqua representing prevalent issues in our clan. I'd like to think, that awareness will make the intergenerational toxins less potent for them. (Hautman Bates, 2014)

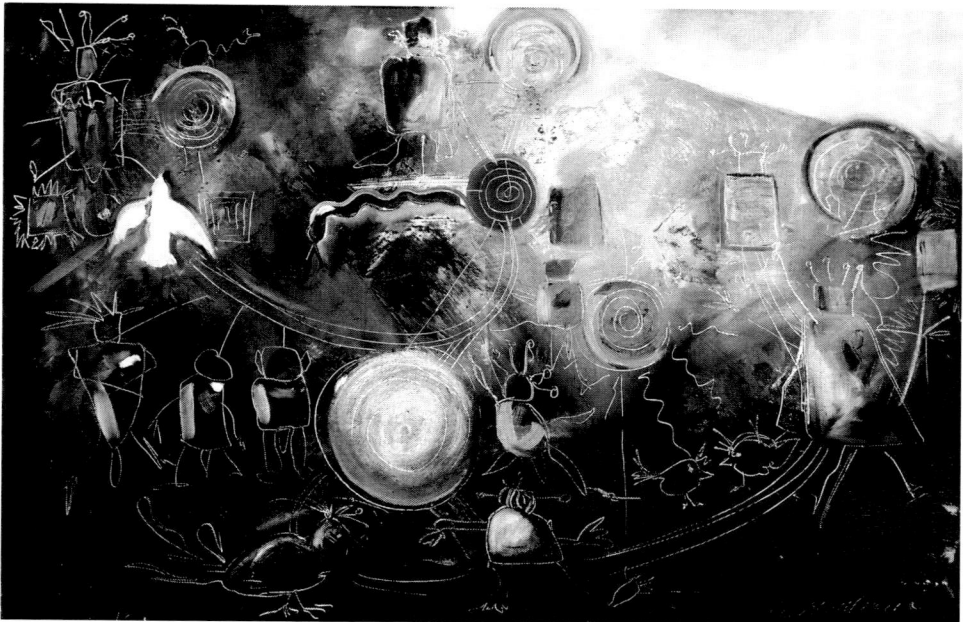

Figure 3. Oil Painting Genogram, Amy Hautman-Bates.

Every student I've ever taught in my family art therapy courses has been required to create his/her own art-based genogram. I don't want therapists to try things with clients that they haven't experienced themselves. And so, year after year, my students let me know that although this creative process often held pain, it has also held enormous meaning for them as they struggled to let their own families become visible.

Christine Kerr, another art therapy educator and family art therapist, spoke of this need for students' self-awareness:

Family art therapy training also needs to address the importance of the family art therapist's self-concepts it relates to the therapeutic alliance with future client families. . . . Family of origin exploration is considered an optimal teaching tool to help the trainees examine the emotional and behavioral patterns of interactions occurring in the family in which the trainee was raised. (Kerr, Hoshino, Sutherland, Parashak, & McCarley, 2008, p. 107)

I invite students, as I invite clients, to choose media and materials that they're pulled toward as they think about this exploration. Students have let their choices speak to their art-making passions, and sometimes to family traditions. Hand-stitched quilts have explained the family ancestors, relationships and patterns (see Figure 4). Recipes and pictures of food (sometimes including samples) have spoken of family values and history shared through food. Food, actually, is often an emo-

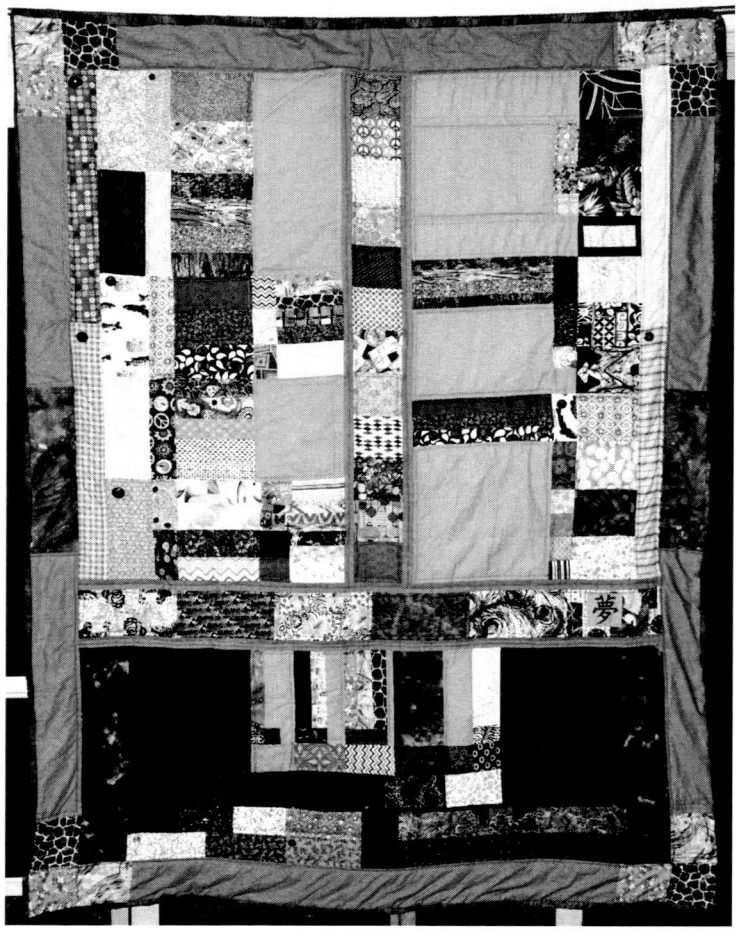

Figure 4. Quilt Genogram, Candace Ayles.

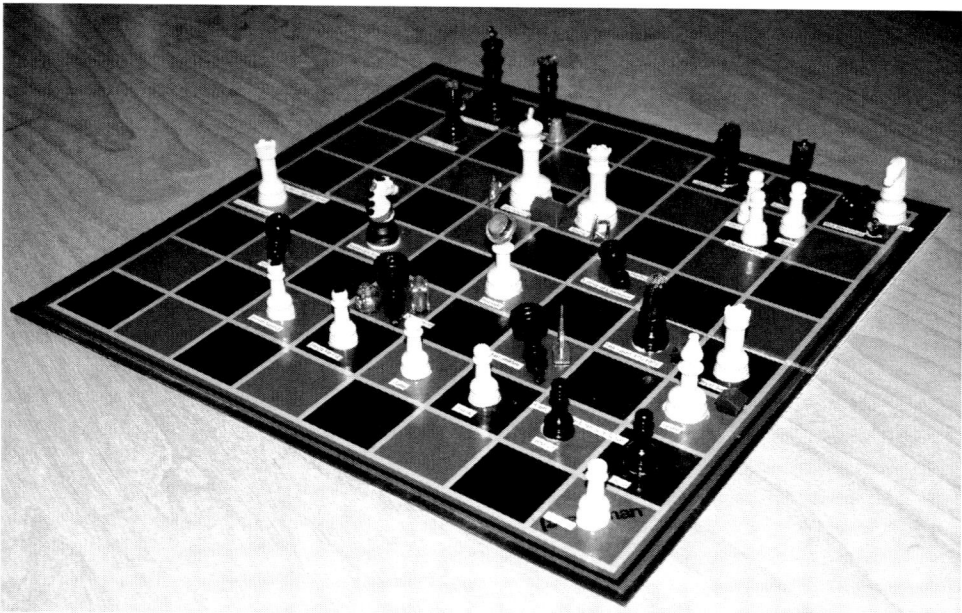

Figure 5. Chess Board Genogram, KaSandra Verett.

tionally charged issue within family of origin work and "food rules," spoken and unspoken are as numerous and complicated as "gender rules," "money rules," and "sex rules."

Family rules were very clearly present when a student used a chessboard as the basis for her genogram (see Figure 5). Roles and rules for behavior became clear as she decorated and embellished the pieces. She had an accompanying print-out of the rules for each piece (or family member). When she finished the complicated description of how her family of origin gave meaning and order to the world, the rigidity of each person's role was very clear, while the nature of the game and game pieces remained. Cathy Moon has written extensively about material choice:

> Materials, particularly those not considered traditional art materials, have hybrid identities. No matter the level of transformation a material undergoes in the process of art making it retains a trace of its former identity and the utilization purposes or functions for which it was intended. These functional characteristics influence the way the material is understood and the response it evokes. (Moon, 2010, p. 68)

22 *Exploring and Developing the Use of Art-Based Genograms*

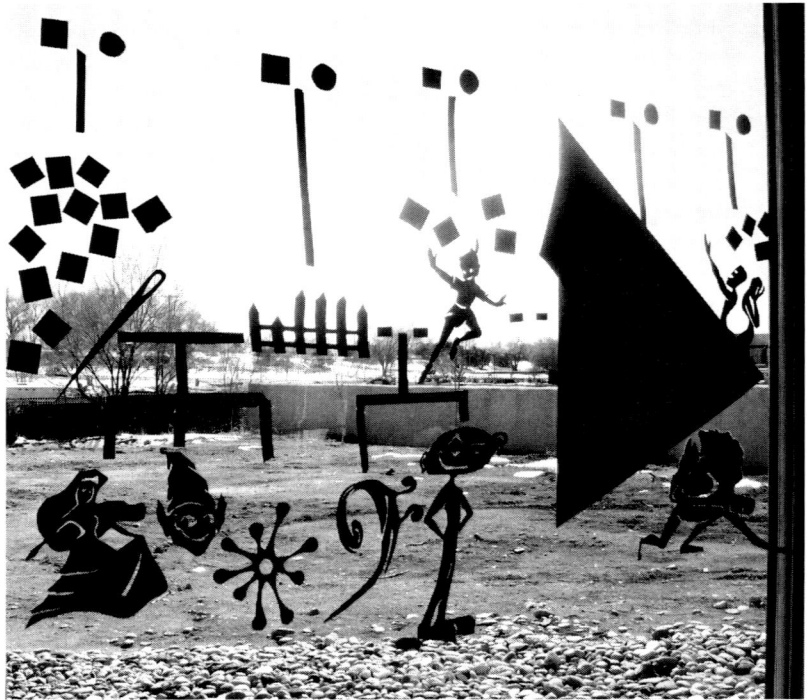

Figure 6. Window Genogram, Kim Douglas.

When one thinks about purposefully evoking the presence of family members in an art-based genogram, it's not surprising that the sensual nature of art making informs material and media choice. When I touch a smooth piece of walnut wood I feel the presence of grandpa Walter who made beautiful decorative pieces out of walnut. Most of us can time-travel through a whiff of a familiar scent. There's a carnation-scented perfume that brings Grandma Martha into the room again for me. Moon acknowledged the power of our sensory responses to materials when she wrote:

> Physical and sensual responses are the core of any interaction between maker and material. . . . Bodily and sensory engagement, in turn, evokes memories and associations to times, places and experiences. (Moon, 2010, p. 61)

A soft tee shirt was utilized by a young mother who used a bleach pen on the dark material. She reversed the usual order or structure of the genogram, starting with symbols for grandparents at the bottom of the shirt, and ending up with her daughter's symbol placed literally over her heart when she wore it.

Several students have created genograms on sections of the art therapy classroom floor, using objects that represent family members, sometimes with yarn or rope creating the connecting lines between people. We watched as the genogram creator moved and stood between and among the representations of family. Often the student was visibly moved by touching and holding the pieces, particularly if an object had actually belonged to the person that it represented. Another student used black paper images that she stuck to the windows of the classroom (see Figure 6). The world outside appeared eerily between the images of family and spoke to the concept of family within the context of the larger world. A rather delicious genogram appeared on the top of a large chocolate cake, with family members created from frosting and candies. The student's peers and I happily helped her eat the art-based genogram, somehow allowing a rather difficult family history to get eaten all up.

This kind of temporary art statement seems reminiscent of the illusive mysticism present in sand paintings – completed only to be present momentarily and then disappear completely. Therapists have used this transitory experience in their work with trays of sand and tiny figurines, as another way of creating genograms. McGoldrick, Gerson and Petry include a chapter entitled "Family Play Genograms" co-authored with Eliana Gil, and within it the value of the use of metaphor is clear in the use of the miniatures in the sand: "The symbolic nature of the miniatures makes them a fascinating tool for drawing out unrecognized family characteristics and patterns in a creative and fanciful format. . . . Projection occurs when clients infuse objects with emotions or personality traits; it creates a safe enough distance in which to begin to acknowledge, understand, or address personal issues" (2008, p. 261).

Author and marriage and family therapist Bonnie Badenoch wrote:

> We frequently ask families to find objects that remind them of each other, always including one for themselves. . . . In one family of four, the parents chose nothing but angry figures – lions, panthers, a raging face, a stern policeman – to represent one another, while the children selected vulnerable baby animals for themselves. . . . Hours of conversation may not have made their situation this clear with such forceful impact. (Badenoch, 2008, p. 227)

When students or clients choose to create genograms that by their very nature will disappear, I ask permission to take photographs. As metaphoric meaning evolves, it feels important to have a reference point that holds the original visual statement. And sometimes the exact opposite art statement is made when students or clients create art-based genograms with an intention of permanence, a strong art statement that is meant to exist for future generations to touch and share. I've witnessed metal sculpture and beautiful jewelry that captured the people and stories within a family, created with heartfelt tenderness that seemed to send a message of love into the future.

Chapter 4

THE VALUE OF HISTORY IN A "HERE AND NOW" CONSCIOUSNESS

During the intensive "Family Weekend" at the residential treatment center, I found myself putting a piece of ice in Kenna's hand. She'd been triggered while listening to her sister talk about a childhood memory and had dissociated a response that had probably been helpful in childhood. Her psyche knew that it could deal with the trigger by going away. The ice cube and my voice helped bring her back into the room, back into her body, and back into the present.

On Sunday of that same weekend, all families were asked to create art-based genograms. After some playful attempts at creating an oversized handbag to represent a "goofy aunt," Kenna's family settled in to brainstorm images and symbols. When art-making time was finished, Kenna's mom, Margie, shared quietly about the presence of sadness that she experienced in the genogram. She noted that although in family history the word "depression" was never spoken, the family would worry when great-grandma used to spend a lot of time in her room, or quit answering the phone, or stopped going to church on Sunday. Margie became teary when she talked about her own sadness and the day last fall when she couldn't get out of bed, and when Kenna heard about her mother's experience she began to tentatively believe that her own struggle with depression could perhaps be held by her family in a more open, nonjudgmental way.

The paradox of holding and appreciating past and present is observable in multiple facets of daily life. People sign up on internet sites that help them find out who and where their ancestors came from, and some have their DNA tested for the scientific clues. At the same time they take up meditating, yoga and reading Eckhart Tolle to more fully engage in awareness of the here and now.

As reimbursement and health insurance issues swirl around the mental health field, clinicians can be encouraged to work more quickly. Rumors of "how many sessions" we can get paid for push us to be more concerned with finding solutions for today's problem very quickly, and sometimes that's completely appropriate. I remember a client who came to therapy after ending an abusive relationship. She was exhausted and shaken, scared about what her young children had witnessed. We initially talked about resources, support systems, and being safe. It wasn't the time to go deeper. Eventually, we did use art to explore family of origin issues, and there was a pattern of women and men in physically abusive relationships.

Long before I went back to college to study art therapy, I went to my first therapist. I was terrified of the panic attacks that I was having, and I desperately wanted them to stop. And after a few months of therapy they mostly stopped. Anxiety transports one to the future, and I had to learn how to tolerate the symptoms in the present and manage stress in a different way. Years later it became possible for me to look at the origins of all that anxiety.

A key issue that separates the unhelpful time travel into one's past and focused family of origin work is intentionality. If one is unwillingly hijacked by a triggering smell or voice, back into the past, we work hard in therapy to develop a tolerance for discomfort and an ability to stay grounded in the present. It feels very different to use art making to bring back an evocative relationship that helps one connect with one's past in order to understand the choices impacting the present and the future.

On a rare rainy evening in Santa Fe I found myself pulled to an art show and lecture by international travel writer Judith Fein. When this small dynamo of a woman began to speak I knew that I was in the right spot. She spoke about the travels and relationships that led to the writing of her book *The Spoon from Minkowitz: A Bittersweet Roots Journey to Ancestral Lands*. She also spoke about the art making she did, following this ancestral journey, and so I bought her book and immediately began reading. She used a phrase that completely resonated with me: "emotional genealogy." I contacted her after finishing her book and share her words here:

DS: Can you speak a little more about the idea of "emotional genealogy?"

JF: Emotional genealogy has three components. First, is learning family stories. The best place to start is with the oldest family members – grandparents, aunts and uncles, cousins. Most people have never asked. The second component is tracing family behavioral traits. Once you understand them, it gives you a choice about transforming them so you don't have to transmit them. And the third component is Knowledge in the Bones – places and groups of people you are attracted to, countries that fascinate you. Often there is a real link to those people and places. All three of these components help you to understand where you come from, who came before you, and what has been passed down to you. Whether you do this exploration or not, your ancestors continue to impact almost every aspect of your life. If you do the exploration, it opens up a world of choices. In my book, *The Spoon from Minkowitz: A Bittersweet Roots Journey to Ancestral Lands*, I invite the reader to come with me as I connect the dots of my life. I hope that when they see how my world opened up based on six tiny facts I learned, it will encourage them to start looking into their own lives and how they have been impacted by their ancestors and the past.

DS: How has your journey into your family's past, helped or healed or informed your present?

JF: It has opened my heart to gratitude, and to understanding what my ancestors endured so that I could live and flourish. It has given me a sense of rootedness that stands in stark contrast to the rootlessness of many people in America. They hardly know their grandparents' names, or where the immigrants in their families came from. I feel connected across time and space. I know where I come from, so I know who I am.

DS: Could you speak a little about your own creative expression following your journey, and why it was important to incorporate the art show into the discussion of your book?

JF: I became so involved in ancestors (not genealogy, not names and dates, but the aspects of emotional genealogy), that I was stunned, while I was on assignment as a journalist at Ted Turner's ranch, to realize that animals had ancestors too. I started collecting bison and elk bones, and I began to do art with the bones. Each bone "spoke" to me and told me what it wanted to become. Through this form of creativity, I made works of art that connected me to my past, my grandparents, my great-grandparents. I realized you can access and express your past through art, as well as through words (personal communication, March 11, 2014).

The art on the walls and tables that evening when Judith spoke, was moving and powerful. Artists shared their memories and stories through their art and I felt the goodness and health present in this honoring of people who came before. So many people in the audience had lost family members during the Holocaust and there seemed to be a yearning for the kind of information and experiences that Judith shared from her travels in the Ukraine.

Ruby Gibson is a somatic therapist and earth-centered ceremonialist who has specialized in healing generational suffering through a practice that she developed called Somatic Archeology. She believes that our bodies hold family patterns and memories that go back seven generations. She traces this belief spiritually to the concept that Iroquois Chiefs considered how their decisions would impact the next seven generations (Gibson, 2008, p. 43).

She stated:

> Ancestral memories are designed around the need to perpetuate healing and pass forward the wisdom and recklessness of your forbearers (p. 48). She developed a method and steps for 'excavating' and eventually healing familial and ancestral traumas and sorrows. She believes that not only do our bodies hold the somatic memories of seven generations of ancestors but that our current actions and behaviors affect seven generations into the future. "Therefore, what you heal in the present time you are also healing backward, forward, and horizontally, affecting your ancestors, your children, your great-grandchildren, your immediate family circle, and your tribe or community. (p. 43)

I must admit that I don't have a cultural or spiritual context that truly holds the idea of healing backward, or healing the ancestors, except perhaps in the power of understanding and peace that I can bring to the past. And that can most certainly impact choices affecting current life and the lives of future generations.

A facet of Gibson's work deeply resonates with me as an art therapist. She spoke of collective memories as being primarily symbolic, visible understandings of invisible concepts. "Deeply mythological and prophetic, symbols, totems, glyphs, and artwork are the messengers of the spirit world" (Gibson, 2008, p. 43). A concept eloquently shared by one of the leading authors in the field of art therapy, Shaun McNiff, who wrote:

> If we imagine paintings as a host of guides, messengers, guardians, friends, helpers, protectors, familiars, shamans, intermediaries, visitors, agents, emanations, influences, and other psychic functionaries, we have stepped outside the frame of positive science and into the archetypal mainstream of poetic and visionary contemplation. (McNiff, 1992, p. 74)

This idea of image/art as messenger is particularly appealing to me as I think of an art-based exploration of ancestral beliefs. McNiff stated: "Even the most unmystical art therapist approaches paintings as messengers from the inner world" (p. 76). It is in this spirit, believing in the almost magical truth of art's messages, that I invite the symbols, the metaphors, the art, and the archetypes into art-based genograms.

Dr. Thom Allena, a community and organizational psychologist, is well known for using an archetypal sensitivity in his work with conflict transformation and restorative justice. I was intrigued when I heard about his work that so often involves the personal and collective histories of communities, and he graciously agreed to talk with me about his experiences. His work with restorative justice mirrors many of the words that I use when I talk about the healing process with families. He speaks of the role of metaphor, images, memory, places and performances. He speaks of "transforming historical harms through (1) facing history, (2) making connections, (3) healing wounds, and (4) taking action."

In speaking with him I felt a resonance between his healing processes and the advocacy and social justice work undertaken by art therapists for community empowerment and healing. He uses "Restorative Circles" with communities that have experienced violent crime or traumatic wounding. This method of restorative justice comes out of indigenous communities and First Nation Circle Work.

He emphasized the idea that all members of the community have an opportunity to share their own experiences which moves the process away from contemporary punitive justice that focuses on the offender, toward community members sharing their narratives and eventually creating an opening where understanding and even compassion can exist. He asks: "How do we repair the harm to the victim? How do you restore balance in the community? And how do you have those that offend make different choices in the future?"

Although he works nationally, we spoke specifically about New Mexico since this was the location of our discussion. He spoke of New Mexico's 400-year history of unbroken trauma and stated that "There are enormous shadows here." I asked him what the symptoms of trauma are in institutions and communities and he listed: "Denial – we aren't going to talk about it, scapegoating, anger blame, violence and addictions" – issues that we read about daily and experience personally here in our "Land of Enchantment" and certainly also on a national level. This beautiful state with much true enchantment, exists much like our clients who have repressed lives of trauma and abuse. There can be no denying the effects of colonization and waves of violence within this landscape.

Allena values the landscape as a container for history and speaks of "Terra Psychology." In his teaching at the University of New Mexico, he asks his students to spend time on the landscape and reflect on the narratives that they're hearing from the land. Then he encourages them to respond in metaphor, using art, poetry, song, and so forth. Allena asks us to consider whether places might carry the visceral remnants of violation. He speaks of animated phenomena associated with places in New Mexico, social violations and terra firma reconciliation. He believes that the intergenerational transmission process passes unconscious tasks on to future generations. In other words, if we don't deal with it, the next generation will. A wider view of what we know about family work, and the importance of moving forward informed by our ancestors; feeling the freedom to make healthy choices (personal communication, Nov. 24, 2014).

During our conversation I was reminded of the many times my colleague Dr. Carol Parker has spoken about the healing within rituals and ceremonies, and her own deep connection to the land. A wilderness guide and shamanic practitioner, she agreed to talk with me about her beliefs:

> Our indigenous elders and healers tell us that ancestors can get stuck on the earth plane after passing. This may be due to a traumatic and unexpected death in which the soul is unprepared for the sudden passage into Spirit. Or it might be that the ancestor had no one available to do the traditional ceremonies to help the soul pass into higher realms. In our Western culture, we are familiar with the possibility that a place or house might be "haunted." Similarly, the site of a traumatic event such as an accident, massacre, or natural disaster

can result in a sense that the place is inhabited by distressed, sad, heavy energies.

These heavy energies or "stuck souls" can be cleared with prayer and ceremony. Indigenous medicine people have traditional ceremonies and prayers for this purpose, passed down through the ages. A modern person, trained in shamanic techniques, can perform a ceremony they have learned, or can simply employ powerful prayers from tradition. Oftentimes, a plant such as ceremonial tobacco (nicotiana rustica) grown for noncommercial use is a highly powerful ally when clearing ancestral energies from a place. Traditionally the tobacco would be prayed over, then smoked in a pipe or cigarette; the smoke from the tobacco plus the prayers help clear the site and help the souls move to a higher level or "towards the Light" as some medicine people describe it.

The land itself does not "hang on to" these energies. Mother Earth doesn't cling to these energies. However, accumulated energies in a place on earth can create a sense of "heaviness" or sadness. We have all had that sensation, for example, at a war memorial, or at a place where many people were massacred, or perhaps in someone's home where someone has died recently. It is up to those living on earth to clear these areas as quickly as possible.

About four years ago I made a traditional pilgrimage in the Apennine Mountains of Italy, along a route walked by thousands of Catholics over the centuries. These Catholics each carried (and still do), a huge stone up the mountain as penance for their sins. At the top of the mountain, they deposit the stones in a heap, then depart from the site feeling unburdened. When I arrived at the site, I felt almost ill from the accumulated heavy emotions and energy of the place. It felt awful!! It was then I realized that the Catholic tradition does not emphasize clearing these energies. The ceremony of hauling stones up the mountain in penance was only half complete . . . the other half was to employ ritual, prayer, tobacco, incense and other known methods to release all the heaviness. These heavy energies, whatever their origin, need to be cleared as quickly as possible.

Eventually, heavy energies from trauma, sudden death, or whatever the human source, will leave the earth plane. New forests will grow over old sites, haunted houses will be torn down, confused souls will finally move on. However, these energies don't have to linger. We can learn the "old ways" of clearing and cleansing. This is important so that the suffering of the ancestors is healed and what gets passed forward to our children is joy and health. (personal communication, Dec. 29, 2014)

Passing joy and health forward to our children, feels to me to be the sweetest gift that we can give. And therapists can help people uncover this gift which may have been buried, in some families, for many generations.

Chapter 5

THERAPEUTIC USES IN INDIVIDUAL THERAPY

I like to think of an art-based genogram as a living image, one that we can create in therapy and then follow as a treatment planning tool. As the image develops and some clarity forms around the nature of relationships, we may veer off and encourage another art response to the art that is present within it. Ellen's story exemplifies that kind of fluid use in individual therapy. Ellen's light gray suit was impeccable. She appeared as polished and professional as ever but I noted that the circles under her eyes seemed particularly dark. I asked how she'd been sleeping. This little question was answered with tears.

In her early forties, Ellen had recently gone through a divorce and had sought therapy for the sadness that wouldn't leave. She had hoped to move through the divorce and aftermath with the same efficiency that fueled her work day. We'd recently been playing with the idea of tolerating mess by engaging with slightly messy art materials (her suits always well-protected with an art-shirt). A "failed marriage" seemed to be the first visible "mess" in her life story. She'd willingly created a visual timeline with collage images that reflected only success until the divorce. Success in high school sports, success in college with impressive grades, success in landing a promising job and the subsequent moving up the career ladder, success in finding a "perfect" husband, and success in giving birth to twin daughters.

I was curious to find out where the absolute black and white beliefs around success and failure had come from. "The absoluteness of perfectionism does not provide for repair. There are only two categories for people: perfect and imperfect. . . . A strike against you is a strike against you forever" (Fossum & Mason, 1986, p. 25). I talked with her about the idea of creating an art-based genogram. She seemed a little dismissive of the idea that generational family beliefs might have anything to do with her current experience, but she agreed to give it a try.

She began by creating images for her maternal grandparents. She used oil pastels and quickly drew a gavel to represent her grandfather who had been a judge and then drew a teapot for her grandmother whose life seemed to reflect a penchant for numerous social engagements. When she tried to create a line between the two images indicating their long marriage, the oil pastel line turned out wobbly-looking. Unable to erase, Ellen worked on another line right next to the first one but it smeared. Clearly frustrated, she said "They had a long marriage! We don't believe in divorce!" I love the honesty of the art-making process.

As work on her genogram continues, it was clear that the image representing her grandmother and the connecting lines to and from her grandmother held a particular charge. In imagery it's easy to spot areas of visual power. Her grandfather had literally held the gavel and role of judge in life, but her grandmother had carried the judgmental voice of the family.

I invited Ellen to amplify her image of her grandmother by using a technique with an art therapy assessment, the Family Centered Circle Drawing. Developed by Robert C. Burns, the purpose of this art therapy assessment was to understand parent-self relationships (Brooke, 2004, p. 90). I modified the assessment to simply focus on Ellen's emotionally-charged image of her grandmother.

I gave Ellen a piece of paper with a circle, about the size of a dinner plate, already drawn on it. I asked her to create an image of her grandmother in the center of the circle, and then draw symbols that she associated with her grandmother, around the outside of the circle. Ellen said "I don't know how to draw people" but began sketching in an oval face with pointy-tipped glasses. The mouth was a straight line. She didn't draw her grandmother's whole body, stopping at around the shoulders. She colored in a white tailored blouse and pearls, "She dressed up every day." I smiled and expressed wonder at being able to do any housework or child-rearing while all "dressed up." "No, there was a maid," was Ellen's response. Symbols that appeared around the outside of the circle included a musical note, a deck of cards and a brown rectangle that was later identified as a meatloaf. As Ellen began talking about the symbols, it became clear that they were intertwined with memories of Saturday evenings in childhood. "We went to our grandparents' house almost every weekend, often for dinner on Saturdays. I remember my parents arguing on the way over, but I don't remember what it was about."

She pointed to the musical note. "Playing an instrument was a requirement in my family. I would bring my sheet music with me and play a few pieces on my grandmother's piano. Always classical. I tried playing a Beatles song once and was asked to play 'real music.'" Ellen smiled when I gestured toward the brown rectangle. "Meat loaf. Almost always meat loaf, potatoes, canned green beans, and Jello with Cool Whip." I asked what it was like during those dinners. "Horrible. My brother and I would be watched for our manners and one of us would always mess up. And I don't think that my grandparents like my dad. There were sarcastic remarks about things like politics and other people. But the worst part was after the dishes were done and the cards were brought out."

"Playing cards was the worst part?" I asked. Ellen went on to describe games of Hearts and Rummy that were brutally competitive. "It wasn't play. I'd try so hard to remember what cards other people had played and I couldn't do it. Sometimes my uncle would try to cheat and if he was caught he's get beet-red in the face and throw down his cards and leave the table. My grandmother usually won, but grandfather and dad won sometimes. Winning was important."

Over the next few sessions we explored the family members associated with winning and success. In her genogram Ellen represented her mother as a house. She'd been a homemaker when Ellen was growing up and later became a realtor. Ellen remembered being grilled after school, about her day. Only "As" were allowed and blue ribbons were expected. Each season involved a sport and any losses were discussed at length. Visually, the genogram seemed tight and rigid, the lines connecting people reminded me of a spider's web. Ellen seemed to stop breathing when she sat with it, and I asked her if there was any place that felt more open or easy within the visual image of family. Her shoulders relaxed when she pointed to Aunt Chloe, her dad's sister.

"She and my dad always joked around a lot and I think he missed her when she moved away." Chloe was a chicken in the genogram. "She has chickens, really, she does! In her backyard." Ellen seemed happily amused when sharing stories about this aunt who broke many family rules and traditions – and paid the consequences for "being different." Bowen spoke to this dilemma that family members may experience when moving toward differentiation. The message from the family is essentially "You are wrong . . . change back . . . and if you do not, these are the consequences" (Bowen, 1978, p. 495). Gibson, also speaking to the possible consequences of one's healing work stated: "Healing your story sometimes can be threatening. . . . The significant others in your life may not recognize what is happening inside you" (Gibson, 2008, p. 214).

So, young Ellen heard the comments about Chloe during those Saturday dinners, experienced her own discomfort when having a manners "slip" or a bad play at cards, and absorbed the knowledge early on, about what happens to an imperfect kid or a nonconformist in her family. Ellen's family fits what Fossum and Mason (1986) describe as a "fairytale family" – a family that takes on some kind of socially-accepted person that appears appropriate, successful and healthy.

On the outside, these families are often the envy of others in the community. They live and "act as if" life, that is, they act as if there is a prescribed way for families to live life. . . . The message is implicit yet strong: "If you live life by our rules, then all will be well" (Fossum & Mason, 1986, p. 25).

The mature Ellen eventually sought out her chicken-farming aunt for moral support and was delighted at her own daughters' responses to their "different aunt." The long-term, larger message held by her genogram was eventually a message of hope, anchored in choice. "Perfect" was an illusory choice, and divorce, sadness, and doing absolutely nothing on a summer afternoon, could be present in this new family picture.

"Perfect," upon any mature reflection, might be intellectually known as an illusion, but I listened, and saw in clients' imagery, how it whispers as a subtle yearning. Although we can laugh at the absurdity of a "perfect holiday," a "perfect wedding," or a "perfect spouse," I've seen the concept of perfect seep through the perceived imperfections that sometimes bring people to therapy.

Ivy Ann came to art therapy to explore her frustration at work and to figure out why a job that she had previously enjoyed had turned into something that she dreaded going back to on Monday morning. Sundays were spent numbing out with movies while an "uneasy feeling" grew steadily throughout the afternoon and evening. I invited her to create an image that would help me understand what work was like. She found some glossy magazines and quickly cut out pictures of vases filled with flowers and beautiful furniture. Then she rummaged through some fabric scraps and cut small pieces of interesting, colorful material. She mixed up her images and fabrics together in a collage. She began talking immediately, with passion, about how much fun interior decorating was and the satisfaction she felt when helping customers. This didn't sound like someone who dreaded the beginning of a new work week. I was curious about where my client was in her image, and the room became quiet. "I'm not really in it," she said and with tears in her eyes told the story of a new boss who had her in the back room instead of out front working with customers. Her tears changed to angry weeping and after a little breathing and water, Ivy Ann was able to speak about the indignity of "the back room." The new owner had shifted the percentage of hours spent working with customers and Ivy Ann believed that it was because of her hearing aids and slightly different-sounding speech. The thought of this smart, creative woman being relegated to "the back" of anything was appalling. It wouldn't have initially occurred to me that my client's work-related sadness had anything to do with her hearing loss so I hadn't asked her about it in the intake process.

Ivy Ann had never been to therapy before, and in a later session it became clear that looking at her experience of herself in her family was important. In her genogram, she used pictures of elegant women found in fashion magazines to represent her three sisters and mother. Ivy Ann, a beautiful, elegant woman in her own right, cut out an image of a bear to symbolize herself and said that she never felt good enough, growing up. Knowing that she was "different," she found herself retreating often to her room/cave.

Andrew Soloman speaks eloquently to the differences between vertical identities and horizontal identities in his book *Far From the Tree*. He spoke of the vertical transmission of identity as those things we commonly think of as straits, skills, coloring – anything passed through DNA or shared cultural norms (2012).

> Often, however, someone has an inherent or acquired trait that is foreign to his or her parents and must therefore acquire identity from a peer group. This is *horizontal* identity. Such horizontal identities may reflect recessive genes, random mutation, prenatal influences, or values and preferences that a child does not share with his progenitors (p. 2).

Ivy Ann knew of no other person in her family with hearing problems and her parents had encouraged her to function completely within the hearing world. Ivy Ann could remember her mother saying that she "couldn't remember doing anything wrong" when she was pregnant with Ivy Ann. Soloman stated: "It is easier for parents to tolerate the syndromes assigned to nature than those thought to result from nurture, because guilt is reduced for the former category" (p. 21).

Not deaf, Ivy Ann had no experience of Deaf culture, and although communication had been challenging as a young child, the sense of "being different" seemed to be the huge weight that she carried constantly. "There was something wrong with me and I could be helped but I was never absolutely normal in my family's eyes. I look like my mother and my aunt and it doesn't matter. I'm totally different from everyone."

The groups of people who Ivy Ann had connected with were the other artist-types in high school, and in college she found "her people" in art classes. Identifying horizontally with artists gave Ivy Ann membership in a group of people for yet another trait that hadn't shown up in anyone's memory, in family history. Ivy Ann joked about not being understood as an artist in her family either. She felt loved, but loved as someone almost incomprehensible, to her parents. Parents' ideas about who their children will be and how a child may move the family into the future are murky and mysterious and often based on unspoken wishes.

> In the subconscious fantasies that make conception look so alluring, it is often ourselves that we would like to see live forever, not someone with a personality of his own . . . many of us are unprepared for children who present unfamiliar needs. Parenthood abruptly catapults us into a permanent relationship with a stranger, and the more alien the stranger, the stronger the whiff of negativity. (Solomon, 2012, p. 1)

No matter how many statistics that the media shares with the public regarding new trends, methods and styles for parenting, on both an unconscious level, and from a conscious place, people also have fantasies and dreams about how and when, and with whom, their children will appear in their world.

Jordan was frantic about his ability to parent when he came to therapy. A young single father of a two-year-old, he worked at a sporting goods store, attended community college part-time, and had his daughter about half of each week. I wasn't surprised to hear that he was having a horrible time sleeping at night, even though he was exhausted. He'd recently fallen asleep in class a few times and was thinking about dropping out. I'd seen his sister in therapy a few years back and she'd recommended me, but she hadn't told him I was an art therapist and he didn't look too happy when I told him. And since he had a lot to say we didn't make art during that first session.

A few sessions later, after we'd looked at the really good reasons he had for laying awake worrying at night, and explored some simple stress-reducing rituals, he got a little choked-up about the morning he'd had. He lived with his parents and his mom usually helped get his daughter ready for day care. Today his mom was already gone, for an early work meeting. So Jordan had combed through his daughter's hair, parting it and putting in the little barrettes, and apparently it hadn't gone too well. "She's tender-headed. And I was in a hurry. When I dropped her off at day care she was still mad at me." Jordan then shared some of his fears for his daughter, unhappy that he and the mother hadn't had any kind of lasting relationship (although their relationship as parents would certainly be lasting). He had such wonderful intentions for his little girl's life, and fear that bordered on despair about his ability to create the life he wanted for her.

I think that it's very easy to feel isolated in a private turbulent sea of perceived parenting incompetence. I was curious what the family history was in terms of caring for its children, and I was delighted that he agreed to use some art to create his genogram. He chose a weather theme, and let people show up as bright suns, rain clouds, and a few storm clouds with lightning. Overall, this was the sunniest weather scene I'd ever encountered. He used a glittery crayon to connect people who had good relationships and between the glittery lines and beaming yellow suns, we almost needed sunglasses to look at it. Story after story of people caring for one another emerged. Even in the parts of family history where storm clouds appeared, it was clear that this family had a rich history of taking care of its own, and sometimes the child next door, too. Perhaps Jordan could relax at least a little bit, knowing that he had a family with a tradition of wrapping loving arms around one another in support and love. Deep inside he'd always known that, but stress and fear had gotten in the way of memory. The art brought reassurance in, from within his own psyche.

Chapter 6

THERAPEUTIC USES IN COUPLES WORK

As a child, my favorite television show was *Bewitched*. The featured good witch, Samantha, had her share of family problems, including marital struggles because of the very different ways of being in the world; mortal and magical. In my child's mind I couldn't understand why her mortal husband, Darrin, objected to Samantha's use of her magical powers. In those pre-feminist-consciousness-raising days, Samantha valiantly tried to deny who she was in order to fit into her husband's world.

As a therapist I'm sometimes still a little puzzled when I work with two people and at least one of them has denied family history and beliefs in order to be more perfect, somehow, for the partner or spouse. Sometimes the differences are subtle and easily overlooked in the exhilarating beginning of relationship. As external life challenges bring stress, these hidden, unacknowledged differences begin to surface.

Expectations around emotional and physical intimacy are often grounded in layers of family history. At the most simple levels of intimate communication, how we speak to one another and how we touch each other, can point to major differences inherited from families, no matter how vehemently each person has decided to be different from his or her family of origin. Riley appreciated Bowlby's understanding of the importance of early childhood development:

> The part I emphasize, and which I feel directly related to couples work, is an understanding (at least superficially) of touching, holding, and bonding attitudes of the family of origin.... For example, youngsters who are stroked and cuddled bring a far different kinesthetic sense to the marriage bed, than those who have been treated in a different manner. (Riley, 2004, p. 135)

When Carli and Alex were working together on their art-based genogram, I watched a little of their differences in showing affection show up. They were seated side-by-side at a table and Carli would occasionally put her hand on his arm or lean close to him as she drew. Alex didn't seem to consciously reject those moments, but during the session did seem to move in the tiniest of increments away from her. His imagery reflected his almost imperceptible scooting away because his drawings began to travel further into his side of the paper.

> Marriage is something of a dance. There are times when you feel drawn to your loved ones and times when you feel the need to pull back and replenish your sense of autonomy. There's a wide spectrum of "normal" needs in this area – some people have a greater and more frequent need for connection, others for independence. (Gottman & Silver, 1999, p. 92)

When we were looking at their shared image, I offered the observation that Alex's images seemed to be moving away from Carli. "I know," he said. "I needed some space." In subsequent sessions they explored the concept of emotional and physical space, using art. Alex eventually remembered his dad's ability to carve out his own space, using a recliner in the midst of family chaos. He also remembered his mother "touching people all the time" and he grimaced as he described her fussing with his clothes or touching his hair.

"What overt and covert messages did partners receive from their families regarding sexuality? Intimacy? Masculinity? Femininity?" (McGoldrick, Gerson, & Petry, 2008, p. 111). These are terribly important questions in couples work.

Art Therapist Shirley Riley would give each person in a relationship a drawing of a four-poster bed. The art directive involved asking them to each draw who or what else was in the bed with them. "Clients may draw a mother sleeping between the couple, father peering over the headboard, grandparents offering a trundle board, children standing all around, telephones and computers in the bed, lamps on and off (Malchiodi, 2012, p. 419). "The bed image often brings out past histories, generational stories, parental influences, and potent emotions" (p. 419). What Carli had considered simple affectionate gestures, Alex unconsciously interpreted as intrusive. Alex's experiences of his own images and his process of making the images opened up his willingness to looking at other relational memories of parents' and grandparents' behaviors. Gibson spoke about what happens when someone suppresses or forgets where they're from: "Historical amnesia creates inner pressure and external conflict as your soul demands self-expression but your heritage demands compliance" (Gibson, 2008, p. 22).

It's no surprise that unconscious and conscious compliance with one's family's beliefs can fuel the emotional charge present for many couples as they face issues forcefully present in everyday life such as money habits and decisions, child-rearing issues, household chores and leisure time. Sheri and Rick came to therapy to work on "communication issues." I found that this word in couples work can cover a huge variety of other complicated issues. When I asked them to begin an art-based genogram, they had trouble moving beyond choosing what art materials to use. Sheri reached for soft pastels and Rick found colored pencils and when Sheri made some initial marks and blew the excess pastel dust away, some of it landed on Rick's carefully drawn image of a car. Sheri apologized and Rick shook his head, rolled his eyes and said "Don't worry about it." Clearly he wanted her to worry about it.

Although we did, indeed, eventually address communication, including Rick's tendency toward passive-aggressive comments, there emerged in that first session, two radically different ways of being in the world. Sheri described herself as impulsive, fun, someone who lived in the moment and her image of herself was a bird in flight. Rick drew a precise rendition of his car and said that he was at peace when he was in his meticulously maintained car (no coffee cups or fast food wrappers in this auto). He spoke about the order of the garage and as I got to know them it was obvious that there was an order and control present in the kingdom of the garage that wasn't present in the rest of their house, or life together.

As their genogram grew, images of their parents showed that they each came from people who valued planning, order, and structure. Rick embraced his family of origin's thoughtful approach to life, and I would guess that initially Sheri felt attracted to what must have seemed comfortable. But her process of moving through adolescence and into adulthood had been to live in reaction to that kind of order and her spur-of-the-moment liveliness, a breath of fresh air at first, had become difficult for Rick to appreciate on a daily basis. "As typically happens, the very qualities that each partner complains of in the other are those that attracted them to each other to begin with" (Lerner, 1985, p. 49).

As much as couples often want us to address the content of their daily struggles (who does the laundry, why there wasn't food in the fridge, and when the last time the floor was mopped), it feels more effective to guide art making and discussion to the issues underneath. In a later session we played a little with the initial genogram images. I asked Sheri to describe what might happen when a bird is trapped in a garage. I asked Rick to describe what it's like to drive Sheri's cluttered car. Underneath the descriptive words that included scared, panicked, uncomfortable and irritated, there was a shared theme of anxiety.

Shared anxiety was almost an overwhelming force in the room when I met Naomi and Tyler. Body language and facial expressions were speaking volumes about the discomfort both seemed to be experiencing. They were coming in following a "boating weekend incident." I thought I'd heard incorrectly when Naomi called. "Boating" is something I never think of in New Mexico. I know it happens but I live in a part of the state where it takes serious intention to see any body of water. When I lived in Wisconsin, long three-day weekends often involved lake activities and the combination of alcohol, sunshine, and lots of time on the boat or beach, did sometimes result in business for therapists the next week.

The "boating incident" turned out to be truly about the need for more honest sharing of feelings and not so much about anything that took place on the boat. Married not quite a year, they had experienced what they considered their first "fight" and it had terrified them both. As I got to know them I asked what their arguments were usually like – how did they disagree, what did it sound like? "We don't" was the emphatic reply, in unison. My bewilderment must have shown clearly on my face and Tyler spoke up: "We don't argue. We believe in talking and compromise." I agreed that talking and compromise are both good things, but surely they each must get a little angry, or at least annoyed, now and then? Naomi spoke: "We never argue. Never. That's why Saturday was so unsettling," and she began to cry.

Apparently on Saturday, driving back from the lake, the tired, sunburned couple had different ideas about what should happen on Sunday. Tyler assumed that they would be back on the boat because his whole family was doing a boating weekend together. Naomi thought that one day was enough and had different ideas for Sunday. And what happened next was like an unforeseen tornado – they yelled at each other!

Both had brought an interesting sense of what being a happy couple should look like, into the marriage, and neither vision contained any room for angry outbursts. While I appreciate setting a line that one does not cross in anger in relationships (perhaps no swearing, no name calling, no insults), I know of no couple who maintains happiness because they deny the existence of anger. This strong aversion to anger pointed to some questions about each person's family of origin. Authors Weeks and Fife believe in the use of the Feelings Genogram:

> Questions about how feelings were handled in the family, which feelings were acceptable or not acceptable, and how different feelings were expressed elucidate the historical basis of these attitudes. Partners can then begin to see how certain feelings were blocked, forbidden, encouraged, or supported. (2014, p. 223)

Weeks and Fife have developed a list of questions that help couples look at their experiences of dominant feelings and emotions in family life. They include questions regarding which feelings were expressed most often and which feelings were unacceptable or not allowed (p. 224).

Naomi and Tyler's art-based genogram provided some important information about the beliefs that each had developed about anger. Naomi's symbols for her parents were swirling red fireballs. She remembered them yelling "all the time" and had consequently vowed to be just the opposite when she grew up. Weeks and Fife spoke of what can happen when anger has pervaded the client's family system: "As a child, this individual witnessed how anger got out of control and how members of the family got hurt. In an effort to never repeat this pattern, the adult partner tries to suppress anger" (2014, p. 133).

Tyler's images of his parents were very different; his mother was a ball of yarn with knitting needles, and his father was a happy face. Tyler said that "voices were never raised" in his family. I wondered out loud how he knew anyone was angry, and his answer definitely painted a colder, quieter version of anger that was about "a tone" or sometimes sarcastic comments. It was hard for Tyler to name these exchanges as "anger." He preferred to dismiss the idea that anger was ever expressed. It took time and some bravery to share family experiences that he now could name as angry exchanges.

> It is not easy to give up the fixed notions that we have about our family. . . . In addition, we may not want to openly ask questions about

taboo subjects in our family. . . . The problem is that when we are low on facts, and when important issues stay underground, we are high on fantasy and emotionality – anger included. We are more vulnerable to having intense reactions to any of the inevitable stresses that life brings – and to get stuck in them. (Lerner, 1985, p. 216)

As we continued our work together, it seemed important for Tyler and Naomi to determine their own way of expressing emotions, and in terms of anger, each decided to take small steps that really were about honesty and authentic communication. Using the statement "I feel" wasn't a simple exercise by any means, when it involved expressing any kind of displeasure. It became a part of creating together, the way that they wanted their marriage, their partnership, to be in the world. It feels to me very much like what Gottman described as "developing a culture:"

Usually when we think of culture, we think in terms of large ethnic groups or even countries where particular customs and cuisine prevail. But a culture can also be created by just two people who have agreed to share their lives. In essence, each couple and each family create its own microculture. (1999, p. 244)

Naomi and Tyler's "boat incident" led to a rich exploration of their families of origin and their intentional efforts to define for themselves, how to be a couple.

My friend Ani Tiffany, a licensed marriage and family therapist, is very firm in her beliefs about the value of family of origin work in couples work: "Marriage counseling is really all about family of origin. Until a couple is aware of what they're each bringing in from their families of origin, all the communication skill in the world won't matter" (personal communication, June 11, 2014).

A point in a relationship when family of origin issues seem to surface surreptitiously, is within child-rearing. "When parents' backs are up against the wall and things get difficult, parents literally feel cornered by stress and revert to what they experienced in their families without even thinking about it" (Tiffany, personal communication, June 11, 2014). We've all heard friends (and maybe ourselves) laughingly say "Oh my God I sounded just like my mother (or father)!"

I truly appreciated my client Priscilla's image of herself as a pitcher continuously pouring out water, nurturing her three children and her partner, but not herself. She and her partner Isabella, were seeking therapy to find some peace around recent stressful challenges that had erupted when they moved in together. Authors Singh and Harper write about the issues of blended families and how those issues may be experienced differently by LGBTQQ partners and couples:

> acceptance or rejection by previous partners and children of changes in the gender of new partners (e.g., for 'opposite'-sexed partners who dissolve their relationship, and one partner forms a new relationship with a now same-sex partner) may prove particularly difficult when navigating such issues as custody and parenting. These issues can have an impact on new relationships as well as on the previous relationship. (2012, p. 294)

Isabella loved Priscilla's children and enjoyed spending time with them, and yet a fascinating glimpse into Isabella's feelings slipped out through the art. Priscilla had created images of her children and placed them between her and her partner. Isabella's response was to draw her own image of Priscilla and place that image on the other side of her own self-image, visually having them appear together, side-by-side in the genogram, separate from the children. This image opened the door in therapy to really talking about how to be a couple and how to also live as parents, together in relationship.

As *Bewitched* continued, it was big news when Samantha and Darrin were going to have a baby. Couples work with this television family could have moved gracefully into family therapy as their challenges together continued to blossom.

Chapter 7

THERAPEUTIC USES IN FAMILY WORK

I remember a story about my great-grandmother of Norwegian heritage who lived in South Dakota. The story is that she could walk by a clothing store window, look at the latest fashions, and then go home and sew what she'd seen. This story fascinated me, growing up. My friend Diane and I would get together to have fun creating doll clothes and I would eventually have to resort to gluing and taping mine together. I did manage to learn to sew when I was a little older, but no other woman or man in our family, who I'm aware of, seems to use their creativity to create fashion.

Family stories are one of the treasures that emerge in art-based genograms. Psychologist and author Mary Pipher elaborated on the value: "Stories reveal what a family wants to believe about itself. They say something about the family, about its character, history and virtues" (1996, p. 244). She continued by exploring the different types of family stories, including stories of adventurers, good deeds, founders of the family, cautionary tales and even vacation-disaster stories. My kids used to beg me to tell the story of a particularly awful vacation taken by their aunt Liz, uncle and cousins. It was a drama that included injuries, car problems, a hospital visit and even a tornado.

My interest as a therapist, in bringing family stories to light within a genogram comes from two different kinds of experiences working with families. One experience is the delight that clients can experience when stories of strength, perseverance, and areas of special abilities or interest emerge from the art. One mother, Rhonda, drew her aunt as a basket of herbs and told her family about summer vacations spent walking out in the forest gathering plants with her aunt. Rhonda's sixteen-year-old daughter, who hadn't been speaking much to her parents, started asking questions about this aunt, clearly interested in the story and resonating with the nature-based healing. This was an opening. It didn't solve anything, but it opened the door for some kind of connection again.

I love the moment in family work when a family starts laughing again.

> Humor is one of the most effective ways to detoxify and reframe a situation. Part of the power of triangles, ruts, labels, and rigid patterns is that they make us feel stuck, take the situation too seriously, and lose our sense of humor. A surprising and gently humorous redefinition of a situation, always without sarcasm, may jostle that inflexibility in such a way that the challenge is softened by the element of sharing. (McGoldrick, 2011, p. 343)

A dad once drew a rough little sketch of his brother, as a dolphin. When asked why a dolphin, he did a hilarious impression of his brother "bobbing through life, goofy and friendly, even when he lost his job!" One of the kids who hadn't ever met "the dolphin" observed that his dad seemed like that too, and he looked at his father and said "You don't let bad stuff get to you, either." Pipher believes that therapists tend to skip over the strength-based stories: "therapists have been more interested in damage than recovery. We have missed the stories about people who did surprisingly well under terrible circumstances" (1996, p. 120).

The dolphin in the genogram was married to a candle. As the family shared stories of the candle "who was like a bright light in the dark," my clients started exploring some beliefs that they held regarding having faith and being positive. The idea of being positive seemed distant to them at the moment since they'd recently been worn down by family struggles. Shirley Riley spoke to how the art opened up her understanding of a family's belief system: "The free form of the genogram and use of color to indicate emotional attachment added greatly to their personal statement and gave 'life' to the many persons involved. I could better enter into their world view when I saw the complicated relationships and cultural implications" (2004, p. 37).

I had that same experience as I entered into the worldview of this particular family as they spoke about their images of the dolphin and candle. We played a little with the idea that perhaps they could each try on a little "dolphin" or "candle" during the week ahead, since one of the newly remembered strengths of the extended family was hopeful positivity.

A different therapeutic experience underlies the other reason I encourage the emergence of family stories through the genogram. This kind of experience is when a family tracks pain or trauma generationally. These aren't the genograms filled with bobbing dolphins or steadfast candles. These genograms contain images of alcohol, syringes, devil faces and tornadoes. I don't believe that it's helpful to gloss over or hide the trauma and pain in a family's history.

> Whatever the family is ashamed of must be discussed. . . . We are diminished by living with problems we try not to see. Secrets keep families from dealing with reality. They keep things from changing and make people feel ashamed. Secrets teach people the destructive lesson the certain events cannot be handled. (Pipher, 1996, p. 143)

During the years when I co-facilitated multifamily group therapy on weekends at the residential treatment center, we usually had between four to six families with us each weekend. Each family had an "identified patient" who was in treatment at the facility and the family members came from all over the country to support, confront, reconnect and heal. During the last few years that I was there I insisted on having each family create an art-based genogram together. I can barely describe the resistance to this, at times. I think that the parents of the adult "identified patient" were often painfully aware of trauma and addiction histories and were afraid of letting these stories be heard – or seen, in the images that would emerge. When families could tolerate this discomfort, however, amazing things often happened.

I remember a family that consisted of parents and three young adults, the youngest being the person living at the residential treatment center. The adult kids drew images of themselves and their parents, and each parent created symbols for their own parents, grandparents, siblings, and even cousins. It was a huge image, filled with a wild variety of symbols. At some point, Ted, the family member in treatment, drew a dark cloud over his self-image. He'd drawn a sad-looking dog and now the dog had a dark cloud over it. His sister asked him what it meant and he said alcohol. Silently, without speaking, his parents began drawing dark clouds over the symbols of grandparents, aunts, uncles and cousins. A difficult weather system was made visible and amid tears, the secrets and stories around alcohol abuse were let out. Not in an effort to blame past generations, but in an exploration of how alcoholism had become both normalized, and not talked about. Suddenly Ted wasn't the black sheep (or sad dog) of the family anymore.

Pipher expressed concern regarding any tendency to blame parents in order to explain failures or documenting only family weaknesses within genograms (1996, p. 115). I understand that concern. I don't support blame, but I have found it important to sit with a family's overwhelmingly pain-filled art-based genogram, acknowledging the dark history. Families can mourn the losses, sit with the sadness and hopefully make decisions that can be transformative for future generations. Badenoch stated:

> The beautiful thing about laying groundwork for visceral, multigenerational empathy is that eventually people are able to *compassionately release* – in essence, forgive – their parents and others in a way that deeply frees them from ties of anger, resentment, and hatred, all of which impede brain integration and subtract from well-being. (2008, p. 165)

I remember a family that colored in bright red faces for all of the family members who were scary when angry. The youngest child who was about fifteen clearly said, while studying the genogram "This has to stop."

A pioneer in family art therapy, Helen Landgarten, spoke to what can happen when this kind of difficult material becomes visible through the artwork created by a family. She warned clinicians to "pay heed to the techniques that evoke strong emotions, bring about confrontations, and/or expose family or individual secrets. . . . Nevertheless, the art experience facilitates interactions, an attitude of openness, insight, and the adoption of new skills" (1987, p. 7).

New coping skills in particular, can be crucial for a family to develop in the face of difficult issues and stressful events.

> From a life-cycle perspective, it is important to track family patterns over time, noting especially those transitions at which families tend to be more vulnerable because of the necessary readjustments in relationships. . . . Problems are most likely to appear when there is an interruption or dislocation in the family life cycle. (McGoldrick, 2011, p. 30)

Therapists who work with families can often normalize developmental stages in family life, and help people to understand that it's perfectly natural to experience discomfort around marriages, births, moves across the country or the neighborhood, kids leaving home, and so forth. The unexpected or unpredictable events such as serious illness, death, divorce, can "potentially disturb the balance of a family emotional system and trigger an escalating cycle of anxiety" (Kerr & Bowen, 1988, p. 234). Kerr and Bowen believed that the lower the level of differentiation and ability to adapt, the number and severity of life problems will increase. The number and quality of life events, the quality of the family's emotional support system, and the general level of anxiety present within the family system and surrounding social context, all impact the family's flexibility under stress. When the ability to adapt is inadequate and life problems surface, symptoms emerge (Kerr & Bowen, 1988). "The less adaptive an individual or a family to stress, the more likely that potentially stressful events encountered early in life will exceed the individual's or family's ability to adapt" (p. 235).

An art-based genogram can actually be a point of problem-solving when a family feels debilitated by a crisis. A family facing a beloved grandfather's diagnosis of early-onset Alzheimer's entered therapy as caregiving issues became more pressing and family members' anger and sadness seemed to erupt quickly into sharp, hurtful words. Using their genogram, I invited them to each amplify and elaborate on their own self-images. What were the strong, important qualities present within each person in this family? What other abilities or qualities seemed lacking? Where were areas of support within the extended family? What community resources could then bolster family strengths and skills? Crystal, who was eleven, had taken soft pastels and created a larger, detailed version of her tiny self-symbol which was a "bookworm" (literally a greenish worm reading a book). One of her gifts that she listed next to her lively-looking worm was that she loved writing poetry. She chose to read poetry to her grandfather after school two days a week. Interestingly, the rhythm of the poetry was soothing and it prompted her grandfather to remember and recite lengthy poems that he'd memorized in childhood.

Within the extended family, a cousin who showed up as a pink donut (someone remembered her loving them as a child), couldn't contribute time, but when contacted, happily volunteered a new boyfriend's expertise since he was a social worker and had some helpful information from his network of colleagues.

When a family in crisis opens up to the widest possible understanding of the word "family," a new openness to giving and receiving love is possible. Almost everyone has a memory of an aunt, uncle, or grandma, who was a person that became a family member through relationship, not biology. A wider view of family support offers a wider possibility of hope. In a book of global family wisdom, author Carol Schaeffer shared the stories and truths of the International Council of Thirteen Indigenous Grandmothers:

> The human race and all of nature are really one great family, the Grandmothers remind us. . . . Families must consciously slow down and simplify their lives. . . . When the 'family fire' is not kept burning, our whole social order begins to decay and fall into disorder. The family unit needs to be preserved first, as that is where strength lies during times of change and calamity. Then the strength of each individual family builds up the strength of the whole human race. (2006, p. 148)

Chapter 8

THE DOGGIE GENOGRAM, OR HOW TO WELCOME IN CHILDREN

It's pretty routine to be asked "What do you do?" at a party. When I say "I'm an art therapist," there are two responses that bug me a little: "You do therapy for artists?," and "Oh, you work with kids." Art Therapy is hugely successful for people of all age groups, so I suppose I get a little testy when people think that if I use art, it must be with children. And honestly, I do love doing art therapy with children.

Often our work with a child or children involves some fairly in-depth exploration of family of origin relatives, rules and beliefs. We may see young children along with their family, or we may see a child alone in individual work and need to either metaphorically or physically invite family into the room. I appreciate Gil's sense of openness in terms of the two basic ways of approaching work with children, directive and nondirective: "I believe that the two approaches are equally useful and can be used in an integrated framework, depending on children's unique needs" (Gil, 1994, p. 14).

I use a combination of directive and nondirective art therapy approaches with any age client. When starting out with a child I offer playful variations of getting-to-know-you art, followed by some art-based exploration of the people (and pets) who are important in the child's world. I often ask children to make a picture (or sculpture) of members in their family using animals. This invites metaphor and play into our session in an accessible way, letting children choose who to have show up and what kind of animals they think represents those family members. Sometimes everyone in the family is a different kind of the same animal. Seven-year-old Mattie's image of her family had big dogs, little dogs and an angel-dog with wings representing her grandpa who had recently died. All of the dogs were lined up in a straight line, a frequent response when one asks a child to represent family members. Next we cut out the dog images and arranged them in a simple genogram shape. Although we glued the rest down, the spotted dog that represented her brother, and the poodle in a ballet tutu that represented my little client, were left movable because they needed to move back and forth between the "Mom dog family" and the "Dad dog family." Mattie spoke for her poodle dog, explaining that sometimes she forgot stuff she needed at one house or the other, and that she shared a room with some "Noisy puppies" at her dad's house and didn't have any space for herself.

Bringing together a group of children who do not know each other and who do not feel sure of their places can put a very great strain on the marriage. . . . I would say that one of the biggest strains in a given blended family has to do with the fact that the children do not necessarily reflect the new joy of the spouses. The question is not *if* there will be strains, but what are they going to be and how will they be coped with (Satir, 1972, p. 182).

In the space of one year, Mattie's family life had undergone challenging transitions. Her parents had divorced and her father had married a woman with several small children. Mattie's beloved grandpa had died. The doggy-based genogram seemed particularly charged with energy when Mattie moved the doggies representing her and her brother, back and forth, from one house to the other. A theme of "not having people" emerged during our sessions and eventually we made a box for each home. Mattie decorated the boxes with glitter and special plastic jewels and each parent agreed to help Mattie find the spot where each box could stay safe in each home. During the conversation with Mattie's dad, he seemed to understand that he'd expected Mattie and her brother to kind of magically become "part of the group," joining in easily with his new family members. The box that was placed at dad's home contained a stuffed animal that Mattie (and no one else) could sleep with there. We asked her mom to spray some of her perfume on it. The box that stayed at mom's house became the special place for another art therapy project, a book of memories of her grandfather. She drew another dog-angel to decorate the cover and added pictures and words to it when she wanted to. Although this memory book was initially worked on during art therapy sessions, I appreciate

Debra Linesch's thoughts about the creation of a mourning scrapbook that the whole family contributes to. The book is left open for family members to use: "They can draw pictures, write a few words, copy some lines of poetry. . . . Periodically the family can gather and each person can have an opportunity to talk about what they have contributed" (2000, p. 44).

Malchiodi and Steele have stressed the importance of helping parents understand an important distinction: "Therapists should teach parents the basic difference between grief and traumatic responses" (2008, p. 268). They speak of psychoeducation around the idea that grief is about sadness and longing and that trauma comes from a terrifying experience that takes away a sense of safety and a feeling of power (2008).

When doing family work with families that include very young children, I believe that having art and play present allowed for a therapy space that was genuinely welcoming for all family members. Unfortunately, young children have often been excluded from family therapy, particularly when the therapist doubts the child's ability to interact well verbally. "What most therapists do with young children, instead, is attempt to impose the adult's world on them. When this fails . . . clinicians relegate them to obscure positions in therapy sessions" (Gil, 1994, p. 34).

Although my sense is that the inclusion of younger children in family therapy seems to have grown since Gil made that statement, I want to emphasize the value of more child-friendly techniques when working with the young ones and the adult family members. Gil speaks of the gift of fantasy that young children bring, and their abilities to explore the world through their senses: "To their own detriment, adults (including clinicians) may play reluctantly with children, unable to utilize their once ample imaginations" (1994, p. 36). Therapists have a unique opportunity, in family therapy, to help reintroduce parents to the magical imaginations and playful realms that their children can access with ease. "It is so important to be curious about who your children are, to learn how to play with them, and to encourage their imaginations" (Cozolino, 2006, p. 331).

Gil suggested that adults and children can be viewed as living in separate spheres and that the therapist can help parents and children merge those spheres. I believe that art and creative play and processes can be the juicy place of connection between sphere. Gil states that: "Adults can retrieve some of their earlier thoughts, feelings, sensation, and wonderments" (1994, p. 38), while admitting that some adults move more easily into their earlier sensations and feelings than others.

I usually invite families with children to participate in some kind of playful check-in at the beginning of a session. The "aquarium check-in" involves a sheet of paper that I've drawn a large rectangle on. A blue line near the top indicates water and I invite each family member to use markers or crayons and show us what and where they are in the aquarium today. Fascinating art statements may tell us that twelve-year-old Patti is upset with her parents – she draws herself as a shiny turquoise fish leaping out of the tank. Her seven-year-old brother Joel is an angry shark swimming menacingly close to the surface. Dad draws some kind of catfish, down at the bottom of the tank "cleaning everything up," while mom draws a mermaid holding out fish food. How will the inhabitants of the aquarium co-exist together today in a way that might feel more positive?

Another favorite check-in is based on Virginia Satir's family sculpture work. I invite each family member to create a Play-Doh® sculpture of something that would tell us something about how they're feeling today. Then I ask them to place their creations on or near a piece of paper, representing home. Sometimes a tiny sculpture is placed clear across the room, perhaps on the windowsill looking outside. It's always interesting to note who is where, who can be physically close to someone else, and what the whole sculpture looks like.

Satir stated that if the children in a family were at least four, they would be included in most of the sessions (1983, p. 183). She spoke of certain things that she wanted to do from the beginning of family therapy, including helping family members "recognize that they are individuals and are different from one another (p. 185). She also hoped to help them "communicate with one another more clearly; to say what they see, think, feel; to bring disagreements out into the open" (p. 185).

My experience is that art-making, in particular, contributes to an increased awareness and acknowledgment of each person's individuality. The difference in art self-images, for example, between a mermaid and a shark, are accessible through the externalization in the art process. It would seem easier for a child to describe how the angry shark feels initially, then to use those "I statements" that therapists work toward. The image can often speak more openly than the small person.

This idea is clearly present in Family Puppet Interviews (Gil, 1994). The process has traditionally involved a variety of puppets so that each family member can choose one and the clinician asks the family to "Make up a story with a beginning, a middle, and an end" (p. 47). The family is asked to "let the puppets speak for themselves" (p. 50). The clinician eventually is able to enter the family's puppet world by asking question, being curious and challenging ideas or beliefs held by the puppets/family members. Gil also encourages the filming of these sessions and stated: "Families have often told me how enjoyable and informative it is to observe their story-telling, and that they have had many insights into their own behavior by watching the taped sessions" (p. 50).

My own twist on this is to ask family members to actually create their own puppets, which can be as simple as brown paper bags or more elaborate through the use of socks, air-hardening clay, and fabrics. These puppets can sometimes be called upon to speak to the family's history, and we can let the puppets help move us into an art-based genogram. When a mom's fairy godmother sock puppet described her aunt as a "rotten tomato," it seemed organic, no pun intended, to ask her to draw the tomato.

In her book on *Mindfulness-Based Play-Family Therapy*, Higgins-Klein incorporates a "Family History Meeting" into the fourth family session in a four-segment intake process: "Genograms give access to valuable information regarding parents' early histories of attachment and trauma and help parents gain more awareness about how they were parented, which in turn helps them reflect on how they could parent more mindfully than they are currently" (2013, p. 48).

Art Therapist Stephanie Murphy understands the importance of knowing the family members' beliefs about their own history. She may have read an extensive file on the family prior to seeing them the first time, but is still interested in looking at what is shared in family history through art. Stephanie has worked with a number of parentified grandparents — grandparents who have needed to step in and care for grandchildren. In my experience with these families I found that the success of this arrangement often depended on the age and health of the grandparents and the ages and special issues of the children. It's easy to imagine the pain of taking over the care of grandchildren from one's daughter or son. I often heard things like "If I'd done a better job with my daughter she wouldn't have turned out this way and she'd have her own kids." And again, it seems helpful to get a wider view, generationally, about what's led up to this.

Stephanie asked one of her in-home clients to create an art-based genogram:

> I was seeing two clients, Susie, 12, and her brother, Sam, 5. Susie was in the fifth grade and truant on a weekly basis. Sam was in kindergarten, and more often than not, in the principal's office for hitting another child, throwing things or using foul language. I tried many times to see them in their own environment, a small subsidized housing apartment. In the beginning of our work together, both children were intrigued with oil pastels, multi-colored papers, and collage materials. But the novelty wore off quickly and I found the apartment empty at my scheduled visitation, or I was summarily dismissed with the magnetic attraction of Gameboys.
>
> The children were in legal custody of their grandmother, a fifty-something single woman, struggling financially on a housekeeper's meager pay. I knew that the mother of Susie and Sam was using heroine, living on the streets, sometimes gone for weeks at a time. Clearly the children were in the best place available to them. Grandma Joanne was also raising another grandson, 16 years old, and often had other family members bunking in at the little apartment. Joanne was angry and frustrated with the chaos at home, and had difficulties with her job, since every few days she would be called to a school for some behavioral issue of one child or another. She tearfully admitted she needed help with them. I made the decision to work with Joanne on a weekly basis; if the children were emotionally and physically unavailable, I would do the next best thing by helping Joanne create a more stable environment in which they could grow.
>
> In our first session, Joanne and I made a "family map" so we could see a bigger picture. We started with Susie and Sam, and their mother. They had different fathers, absent to them. Their mother also had three other older children from different fathers; Joanne did not know where these children were living. We slowly worked our way back in time and expanded the genogram to Joanne's other children, two sons and another daughter. We identified their partners, multiple for each, and all the children born of these unions. The next level of the map included Joanne herself and her siblings, their partners, and finally to Joanne's parents. Once all the family members were named and drawn in place, Joanne began to identify their characteristics and traits by using different colors and symbols above their names. A black cross indicated people that had died a tragic death. A red "A" signified alcohol abuse; a green "D" noted drug use. The many partners of women were circled with a pink "P," identifying prostitution. Purple

("the bruise color") showed domestic violence and physical abuse between adults and children. Joanne used a light blue color to identify family members who were missing. Her choice of colors and symbols, and the fact that she herself drew the map, pulled her in to a deep level of engagement.

The genogram became a tangle of colors and letters, and it was clear to see patterns of behaviors that spanned back through four generations. It was also evident how alcohol, drug use, prostitution and violence, enmeshed the generations of this family into learned behaviors of extreme dysfunction. As Joanne and I looked at the illustrated truth of her family's roots, she began to sob, and said, "What a @%*# mess! No wonder! My grandchildren have so much to be angry about!"

Joanne's genogram illustrated for her a truth she could no longer deny: how she dealt with the challenges of life was learned behavior from her parents that she unwittingly taught to her children, who passed their poor choices to their children. Because of her new awareness, she became determined to break the entanglements and make changes in her own life, for her own sake, and for the betterment of Susie and Sam. Joanne and I worked together for the next six months on boundary-setting, honesty and forgiveness. I did not see Susie or Sam again, but the progress that Joanne made was sure to be influential. As a therapist I had to trust that the change in one family member would echo out to change the others.

Joanne's genogram gave me a deeper sense of compassion and understanding for the acting-out behaviors of children, the generational patterning that occurs for all of us, and the power of art and illustration to inform in a deep and long-lasting way that talk therapy cannot capture (personal communication, Dec. 14, 2014).

When I think about Higgins-Klein's ideas about "mindful parenting," I am reminded of the core elements of intention and choice, concepts that free us from repeating patterns without conscious knowledge and awareness.

Roberto was surprised when his partner Daniel pointed out that Roberto's representation of his father as a fox, closely resembled their son Nathan's image of himself as a fox in their family's genogram. Nathan was nine and he and his younger brother were furious that the family had recently moved across the country. I asked Roberto to share some memories about his father. "He seemed secretive, like he always had a hidden agenda for all of us growing up." Roberto looked at Nathan: "I never know what you're thinking and then you blow up at me." Daniel leaned forward and interrupted: "Nathan is just a quiet boy! He's nothing like your dad!"

Unfortunately, when a parent feels that a child is very much like another close relative, the parent can unconsciously project his or her failings. "The parent's feelings about this relative can be carried over into a positive or negative relationship with the child. Therapy allows the parent to see how painful relationships, past or present, can be harming the current parent-child relationship, and offers healing" (Higgins-Klein, 2013, p. 49).

Satir gave a clear illustration of this when she wrote about a woman reminded of her first husband by her small son: "every time her four-year-old son would say, 'no,' she had visions of her husband always rebelling. Eventually he went to prison for assaulting someone. So when her young son said 'no' to her, her image was of a person already in prison" (Satir, 1972, p. 183).

I asked Nathan what he was feeling, and with much seriousness he stated that he was "not that quiet." We eventually concluded that there wasn't any secret issue or hidden agenda. Nathan had actually been very vocal about his dislike of their new home. The only hidden issue seemed to be Roberto's guilt in moving everyone because of a job opportunity. And Roberto, who was an extrovert, learned some new ways to connect with his quieter children.

I think that most of us who are parents can admit to some unease when we see a resemblance or perceive a character trait in our child that is a reminder of unpleasant or difficult people in our families. Or perhaps it is simply a reminder of something we aren't pleased about within our own selves. Thinking about the future of the next generation does seem like a good time to take stock of what we choose to pass along to them.

Chapter 9

GROUNDED IN THE DIRT

When Teri signed up to take my Family Art Therapy course, she had already heard that students were required to create their own art-based genograms. In her early fifties, she was interested in seeing what would come up for her since she'd already done personal therapy that included family of origin work. Teri shared: "I had anticipated that the art-based genogram I created of my family would be filled with skeletons in closets, since my family falls under the dysfunctional category like so many families do. I assumed that it was a given that I'd be revisiting old wounds."

And then, weeks before she started working on her genogram she had a dream that changed her plan dramatically:

> My dream was brief. In the dream I was surrounded by dirt. It was the deep brown, rich, fertile soil that you can plant just about anything in. When I asked in the dream . . . what it meant . . . I just heard the word "family." I awakened with the realization that I am here today because my family and ancestors not only survived . . . but they prospered. There was a deep sense of gratitude and awe that I felt and it was clear that my art-based genogram would depict this in some way. What I did not anticipate, was how powerfully healing this approach would be for me. (personal communication, 2013)

And so she began her process, grounded in the deep dark richness of the fertile collective, the history of her family's will to survive. Generations of family who had come before her and who had created a space for her to grow. The garden metaphor became the structure that she created her genogram within (see Figure 7).

The garden was indeed a perfect metaphor for the delightful surprises that she encountered as she gave form to the people who were depicted in it. The strengths that were present, the gifts nurtured in the family soil appeared organically. Teri began the genogram by reaching for rough, brown cardboard, a visually earthy container for the plants and flowers. Her garden contained a beautiful variety of plants and flowers, and interestingly, the family members were represented by the creatures that one might see inhabiting a garden. Birds, ladybugs, frogs, bees, flies – branches of the family took on different garden dweller characteristics.

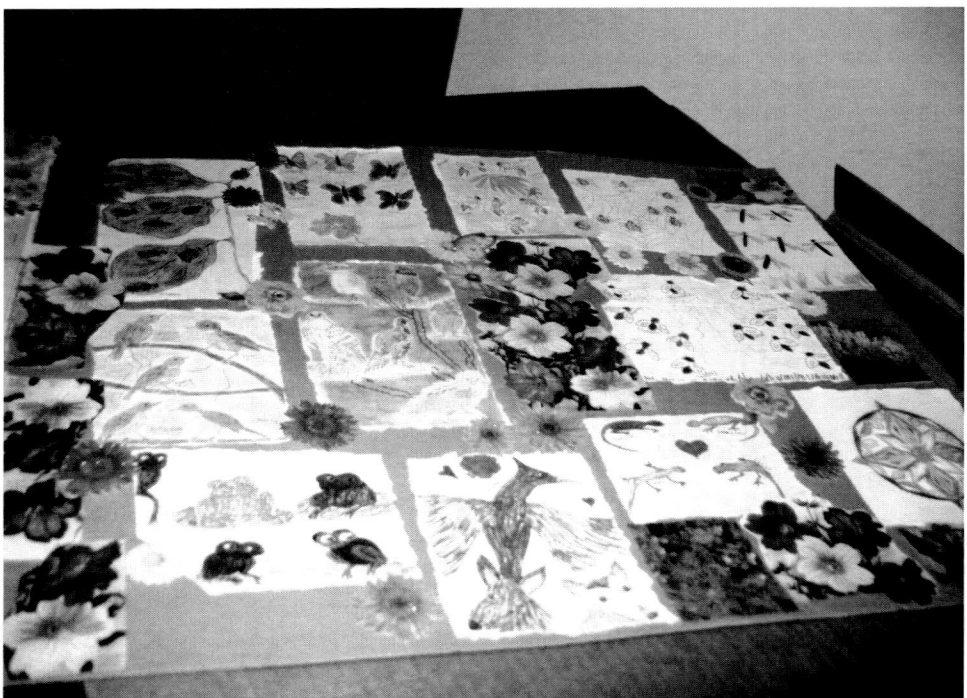

Figure 7. Teri's Genogram.

Teri describes some of the most important garden residents: "My most immediate family members were birds . . . the tyrant flycatcher, falcon, eagle, grouse, and parrot . . . each one carrying a meaning within their names or a connotation that was connected to the type of bird. Although my initial intention was to celebrate and honor family, there were aspects of dysfunction that were evident such as my father being depicted as the 'tyrant flycatcher.'"

Alongside this vibrant garden brimming with flowers and creatures, another art experience developed. It seemed that the collage images of the genogram were actually creating more thoughts that needed space to be creatively expressed. Teri felt the need to record the meanings, values and spiritual underpinnings of her family's ancestors. And so an altered book began to grow, appropriately within an old how-to-garden, loose-leaf book (see Figure 8). "The use of discarded books as an art-making material has gained recent popularity, and it offers the art therapist a readily available, cost-effective material with rich symbolic potential" (Moon, 2010, p. 83). Teri added pages that were cut from the same earthy brown cardboard as her genogram, and on top of the cardboard she used collage to tell the deeper family stories. Stories of countries and cultures, spirituality, and values. Teri shares: "The first pages of this book I used to depict my dream of fertile soil and proceeded with garden images throughout. In the pages I chose to focus on 'gold from the mother line' and 'gold from the father line' as a theme for much of the art. The 'gold' represented gifts bestowed on us from our ancestors."

The strength-based grounding in spiritual beliefs seems particularly important when one looks through this altered book. When I first saw the book I felt that I'd been given a type of key or map to the genogram garden. Teri used collage to pull together the underlying principles that had been handed down from butterflies, birds and frogs, metaphorically.

As Teri explained, both of her parents brought distinct spiritual gifts to the family that she characterized as "gold" within her altered book. Gold became an important symbol, also speaking to the fact that both parents had been the "golden children" of their respective families of origin. When the two "golden children" married, a development of rather grand expectations seemed to arise. The only logical result of two "golden children" marrying must be a rather spectacular family! The artistic task that followed appeared to need some pruning. Teri worked on the idea of cutting away pride, arrogance and unattainable standards as they surfaced in her memories of her family of origin.

The altered book, as guide to her art-based genogram, offers the documentation that supports the growth and challenges of family life. Found within the altered book is a piece of paper saved from Teri's fa-

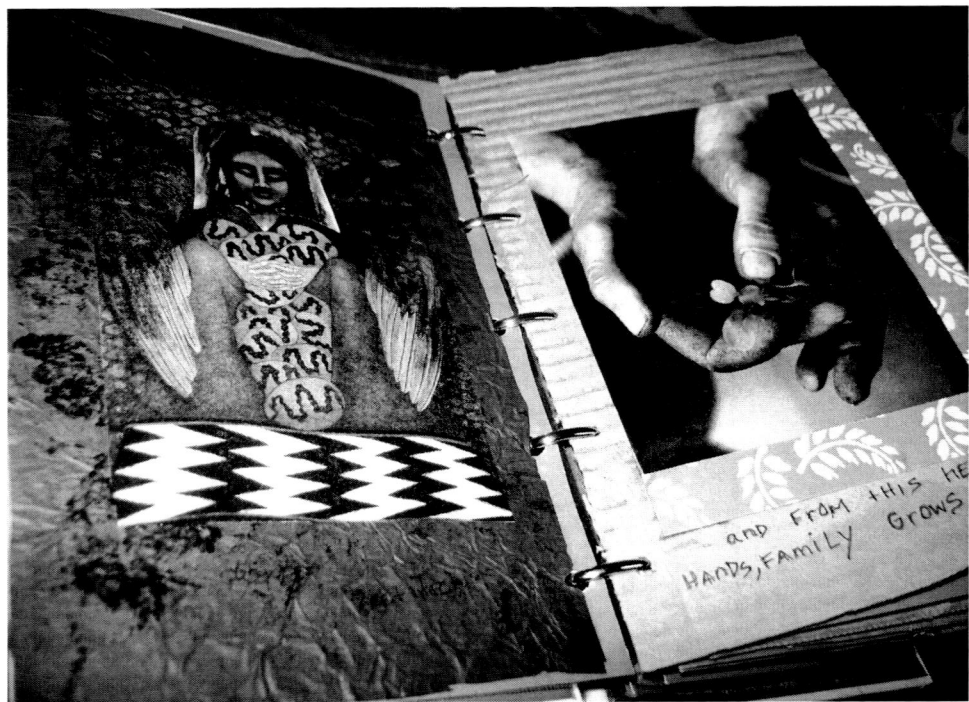

Figure 8. Teri's Altered Book.

ther's funeral. Another small piece of paper surfaced within the genogram itself, a garden poem, well-loved by Teri that her mother used to read to her when she was little. Important little papers collaged into images to enrich both creations.

Because of the unique opportunity for visual expression, a number of strength-based images were given space to be present. Teri was able to let memories show up that spoke to the good we hope families treasure and share with future generations; memories of music, sports, camping, playing cards, and values such as a strong work ethic, and forgiveness.

What a treasure to be able to honor her father's wonderful voice and the presence of music playing inside the home. Teri shared with me that she showed her mother the genogram and the altered book, the next time that her mother visited her. Her mother immediately grasped the importance of the rich soil of the generations of ancestors and was moved by Teri's artistic interpretation of family. Teri talked with me about the healing that happened through the creation of the genogram and book, and the healing that she experienced relationally with her mother. In Teri's own words: "It was a powerfully affirming experience to recognize and celebrate family, and it was very healing for me to do so."

Chapter 10

SAM'S STORY: RIDING A GLACIER

It was difficult for Sam to disconnect from his electronic devices. He wasn't entirely a voluntary client either, and during our first session it seemed to me that he checked his vibrating phone as a way of telling me that his business was more important than the potential of our work together. Unfortunately, the universe had matched him with a therapist who found it easy to turn her phone off and disconnect, and I expect that of others.

Sam was trying therapy at the insistence of his new wife. Married for about a year, she told him that he "only knew how to be angry" and she was unhappy with his apparent coldness and limited emotional expressiveness. She was also concerned about his inability to happily connect with her six-year-old son. Sam's prior marriage had lasted five years and there had been no children.

I wasn't surprised by Sam's sarcasm at the idea of creating an art-based genogram. Because of my absolute faith in the process of art making, I'm pretty immune to objections. When he asked for a regular pencil, I honestly didn't have one. I try to open up the art process by avoiding the precision, perfection and erasure that #2 lead pencils often bring. So he excused himself and went out to his car and brought one in.

With lingering sarcasm he drew a little cube and said that he must be an ice cube. He sketched a triangle that he described as a jagged mountain covered in sheets of ice. This was his father. Above the mountain, several rocks were carefully drawn. These represented his grandfather and a great-uncle, both killed in World War II. He drew his mother as a Christmas tree.

When asked about his relationship with his parents he extended the mountain's ice flow until it touched the little ice cube. "People say I look just like him." When people speak of looking like, or looking nothing like one of their parents, I'm interested in listening for the feelings present around that statement. There is a Japanese folktale about a man who finds a mirror in the street. Totally unfamiliar with mirrors, he believes that he's found a picture of his father, created when his father was a young man. His father had died and so the man treasured the image and hid it away. Eventually his wife found it and believed that it is a picture of a beautiful woman who her husband must be having an affair with. A priest walks by, hears them quarreling and states that they must have been drinking too much wine – the image is clearly that of a priest at the temple (Kronberg & McKissack, 1990). I've always thought that this story has much to share with us when we are tempted to rely on projective art assessments. In the context of family of origin work, there's such important information attached to whether or not one looks like one's parents, and how one feels about it.

Sam went on to say that he didn't really remember if he looked like his dad or not – his dad had died when he was ten. McGoldrick stated: "We all hope that death will occur at a point when family members are at peace with each other and when there is a sense of completion about relationships. . . . Untimely deaths are especially difficult to integrate" (2011, p. 136). I shared some curiosity about the rocks. Sam said "Yeah, it's hard. Men die young in this family. My dad didn't really have time with his dad either."

I asked about the Christmas tree and a brief warmth flickered across his features. "She was all about the holiday when we were little." I asked if he had siblings and he drew a lioness for his stepsister, and his eyes seemed to smile a little when he described her as being younger, but "prowling, watching me, bossing me all the time." As Sam left the session I found myself feeling a little hopeful for the ice cube. Ice starts out as fluid water, and can change.

I was surprised, though, when Sam entered the next session waving an envelope, saying "I brought pictures!" He spread them out on the table. He touched the one on the right and said "I must have been about thirteen. See, there's Susie with that doll she took everywhere." I asked about another picture, a scene at a dining room table with a grinning Susie sitting on a man's lap. He hadn't mentioned his stepfather the week before. Judy Weiser, author and PhotoTherapist, spoke about the value in using family photos:

> When therapy becomes stressful, or there seems to be too much focusing upon the problems rather than the skills clients used to survive their crises, album work can serve as a means of looking at the more positive elements of family life . . . people can be reunited with other components of their lives besides the 'awful' ones brought forward in therapy. (1999, p. 299)

I enthusiastically invited Sam to continue bringing in more family photos as we continued in therapy, suggesting that we could make copies and use them in the genogram.

During our third session together he wanted to add an image of his stepfather but didn't have a picture that seemed to work so he brought out the #2 pencil again and sketched a tiny stick-figure man riding on a tractor. His words caught in his throat as tears appeared. "He was so kind to me. I looked up to him so much. I thought I could be like him with my stepson but I don't know how."

Somewhere in the mysterious growing-up process Sam had felt not quite a part of the new family, and had unconsciously moved toward ice. He showed me a picture of his mom, stepfather and Susie. He'd taken the picture of the happy threesome, and the role of observer seemed comfortable to him in some way. Weiser stated: "In reviewing our personal photographs we learn things about ourselves that we were not at all conscious of when we took the pictures – things that later seem obviously visible were latent or embedded at the moment we captured them" (1999, p. 344).

As our relationship progressed he became more comfortable talking about his father. It seemed as though the language that his father spoke was primarily the language of money, and the pursuit of sports or music or anything that came close to fun, was trivialized. A memory that stood out for Sam was one Christmas Eve when his mom was downstairs wrapping presents and Sam was awakened by this father's harsh anger about how many presents she'd bought.

There were family legends about the frugality of Sam's paternal great-grandparents, but the stories seemed rooted in the poverty of immigrants and survival. "One can sometimes see an intergenerational issue attributable to how things were in their country of origin. Is a family history of famine related to current weight and body image issues? Are present anxiety and trauma symptoms related to fear stemming from past or present immigration or forced migration issues?" (Higgins-Klein, 2013, p. 50). Some small notes of compassion were becoming audible as Sam spoke.

It seemed important, as therapy progressed, to look at the family beliefs frozen in and around the glacier. There were beliefs about working hard, being very careful with money, and the importance of serving one's country. There weren't any verbalized beliefs about men dying young, just some sad facts. Important male authority figures had died young and Sam had no memory of people talking about those sad occurrences.

The eventual thawing of Sam was kind of like spring in Wisconsin. A warm day followed quickly by a light snow flurry. His wife was willing to participate in some couples work and I wasn't surprised to see a few icy patches in her genogram. And I was delighted when she brought in a joyous picture of Sam lifting up his happy stepson at the zoo, pointing out a baby giraffe. "Photographs . . . can help you find out more about what you want from life and where you may be heading" (Weiser, 1999, p. 345).

There were a number of years when I did a lot of in-home family therapy work and one of the huge advantages was being able to see what photographs were hung on the walls. Families often brought out albums and sometimes even home movies, which helped me enable them to develop and share the strengths within their art-based genograms.

I encouraged Sam to spend a little intentional time with his stepfather so he could add some of that kind man's family history to the genogram. Sam reported that visiting with his mom and stepfather and showing that kind of sincere interest opened up new warmth in his relationship with them. As the ice-cube melted, Sam eventually took a (colored!) pencil and drew a small sun peeking out from a cloud as his new way of representing himself.

Chapter 11

ALLIE CELEBRATES PEACH COBBLER

It was so hard to figure out who was who in Allie's story. When there are lots of complicated relationships, or just a significant number of names to keep track of, a genogram is really a perfect way to sort out who everyone is and what their relationships are to one's client. I hadn't heard from Allie in a few years, and she came back to therapy to get a handle on some anxiety symptoms that were flaring up again. The first time that she was in therapy with me she was court-ordered because of mutual restraining-orders between her and her husband. An alcohol-fueled argument had escalated into a harsh physical fight. She had been reluctant at first but quickly came to see the value in taking advantage of "having to come to therapy," and eventually continued on, much longer than she was required to.

That first time around was more crisis-driven. She needed to make hard decisions related to safety and her children's well-being. When the situation had calmed down a little, we worked together to figure out what might help Allie calm down. She worked on self-soothing with watercolor and knitting. She had a delightful sense of humor that had been sharpened over the years as protection from her own hard life story.

This second time around felt very natural to me – we moved back into relationship with ease and she spent some time catching me up on her current life. The kids were doing well, two were out of the house, and she'd moved up the ladder into management at the department store where she worked. She'd divorced the man she'd fought with and life sounded calmer. She developed some solid friendships with people at work, and had dated a little bit over the years. A month ago she met "a really nice man" through a mutual friend and they were seeing each other often. And then she started having some anxiety symptoms that were mild echoes of the panic attacks she used to have.

As she spoke about her wish for this new relationship to be healthy and completely different from past relationships, she began talking faster and faster, spilling out details regarding her relationship history, including marriages, people she had dated in the past and the men who had been abusive to her. Then she started talking about her sisters' partners, her children's boyfriends and girlfriend and a cousin who had been "discovered in Hollywood." It was definitely time to invite art into the room!

I asked her to slow down a little and pick out some art materials so that she could create images representing herself and the new man in her life. She seemed to relax back into the art therapy experience from our prior work together, and drew a sunflower as a symbol for herself. She seemed a little puzzled about creating an image for her new man, and I asked her to just take a minute and think of an image that captured him. What would tell me about him? She smiled and used watercolor pencils to make a picture of a dish of peach cobbler. She touched the image and said: "He's sweet. Really. He's good to me. He's NORMAL." After talking a little about what normal meant to her, I explained the value of the art-based genogram and she agreed to give it a try.

I remembered that her childhood had been almost nonexistent. Her mother used drugs and Allie had run away from home after being sexually abused by yet another man in her mother's life. Imagery appeared of scary mean faces. We had worked a little on her history of sexual abuse in prior therapy, but she hadn't wanted to fully look at that issue before. She hadn't been ready. I trust clients to know when it's time for them to bring such painful issues to light. "Childhood sexual abuse is dangerous. When you were being abused, you may have felt like you were fighting to stay alive. Whether the struggle to survive was literal or metaphorical, fear, terror, and the real or perceived threat of death were visceral experiences for most survivors" (Haines, 2007, p. 184). The anxiety that had resurfaced during this new, safe relationship, seemed linked to the past. "Your body can get caught in a flight, fight, or freeze response, not knowing, on some level, that the abuse is long over" (p. 184). We proceeded very slowly, letting the abusive and subsequent harsh relationships emerge as naturally as possible within the genogram. Angry dark lines connected Allie to the abusers and also to the "wrong-choice men" as she called them.

The negative space where her father's family could have appeared was starkly white in its emptiness. She had no knowledge of this man. I wondered out loud if she remembered any men who had been father figures over the years. Several kind men did show up; an image of a foster-dad during some rare stable teenage years who taught her how to play basketball (so his symbol was a basketball), and a big brown bear appeared, representing a teacher who encouraged her to finish high school. Cozolino spoke about the value of that kind of positive, healthy relationship:

> Loving relationships help our brains to develop, integrate, and remain flexible. Through love we regulate each other's brain chemistry, sense of well-being . . . when the drive to love is thwarted . . . our mental health is compromised. Adults who thrive despite childhood neglect and abuse often describe life-affirming experiences with others who made them feel cared for and worthwhile. (2006, p. 314)

I found it remarkable that Allie had moved forward over the years with so much bravery and strength. "A childhood of sexual abuse does not prepare you well for life. . . . That you survived to adulthood is both a blessing and a challenge. . . . Survivors are very creative people when it comes to staying alive in spite of trauma" (Haines, 2007, p. 227).

One of the gifts that surfaced through her genogram was her pleasure in being a sunflower. No legion of angry faces or fierce creatures had taken away her essence, her positive spirit. As she once again, began some of the activities that she found calming, like walking and knitting, her anxiety symptoms lessened. I think that her ability to deeply believe that she was worth the love of herself and her new boyfriend helped her relax into the new healthy relationship. "If early relationships are problematic, we connect with others in a tentative way, anticipating that what has occurred will happen again" (Cozolino, 2006, p. 322). It takes time to quit waiting for the next bad thing to happen. It takes time to trust that no big bad surprise is around the next corner in relationship. Within this new relationship she found the freedom to relax and be herself. "Learning anything positive, including love, requires freedom from fear" (Cozolino, 2006, p. 322). She could breathe, knowing that she deserved peach cobbler.

Chapter 12

MULTICULTURAL GIFTS AND CHALLENGES REVEALED

The air and energy in the room seemed to crackle and then shift into silence. It was December and the men shrugged off their heavy coats as they approached Evaristo's open coffin. They fell to their knees and began praying the rosary. Sitting next to my partner Joey, Evaristo's son, I had the rare experience of witnessing the *Penitentes*. The *Penitentes*, or *Los Hermanos Penitentes*, are members of a religious society that has kept Hispanic religious traditions alive for hundreds of years.

With deep love, respect and humor, my loved ones and I figure out how to be family while retaining very different racial and cultural ways of being in the world. When we can't figure each other out we can say it out loud. My experience as a therapist reinforced the idea that talking out loud about differences is crucial. And I deeply believe that often, before we can say it out loud, the messages appear within the art and are communicated visually.

Shirley Riley wrote a thoughtful case study (2004) that described the use of art as a way to literally open the door to cultural differences. Anna and Hidalgo came to Riley for marriage counseling, both denying that their completely different cultural backgrounds had anything to do with their difficulties. Riley said: "They were asked to 'draw how it was (in their youth) when one opened the door and entered their family home.' What colors were around? What music was being played? What noise level was heard? How many people were present? Were they talking or being still?" (2004, p. 40). The images they created couldn't have been more different and Riley noted their amazement and the impact this art making had on the couple. "These two had apparently never really *see* their differences" (p. 42). The art moved them from looking for blame or right and wrong and allowed the differences to be present. They were able to illustrate their very different social and cultural realities and see how each other viewed the world (Riley, 2004, p. 42).

Sharing how one views the world is potentially a very complicated, deep process that can be expedited through imagery. Art-based genograms move beyond "multicultural-lite" and allow deep curiosity about family members' understandings of their own people. I think of multicultural-lite as brief visits to any culture that is outside one's own lived experience. These are usually pleasant visits that may involve food, music or shopping. The meaning of the experience may not be visible. I can appreciate the good taste of pinto beans that simmered on the stove all day, and I won't automatically understand the survival stories present in that pot of food. My grandpa, (the garden in my genogram), would buy his cat little treats of Kielbasa (a type of sausage) now and then. The important understanding of that action wasn't about the special sausage. The deeper message was a belief in treasuring those we love, animal or human.

The creation of art-based genograms brings issues of diversity, multiculturalism and even sameness, to life. My clients often were a little surprised by the boldness of ethnic, racial and cultural beliefs that appeared uncensored within the art. Clients said things like "Mom's side of the family was like this" and "Dad's side was like that." "It was fun spending time with dad's family." "I didn't understand what was going on with mom's family." The strengths and difficulties were present and allowed for a gray zone that defied any polarities based on ethnic origins. The loving aunt was pictured as an angel with a threatening fist because she sang in the church choir and insisted on family values, but reinforced those values with physical smacks. The mother of the "hard-fisted angel" was depicted as a stern guard-dog who protected her children during times when the civil rights fight came right up into their front yard. We can welcome the family history into the room through the art and then choose how to honor ancestors and consciously determine one's own behaviors.

My colleague Natalie Carlton and I spent about a week with Navajo therapists and counselors in Arizona. Interested in developing a way of working with families that wasn't necessarily as verbal as traditional therapy, we all worked together, exploring what might be possible through art. We all created art-based genograms and shared them in pairs. As a Navajo therapist and I shared our images, our eyes filled with tears when she showed me the many generations of family members raising sheep and weaving rugs, alongside many early deaths related to alcohol. Gifts present, in the midst of harsh struggles. The Indigenous Grandmothers encourage us to have an openness to our own histories: "We must build on the pain of the past with honesty, even honesty with our children. We can't pretend the suffering did not exist. . . . Only when we give voice to the pain, whether we are the oppressed or the oppressor, can the healing then begin" (Schaefer, 2006, p. 177).

McGoldrick, Gerson and Petry used genograms to explore a number of cultural questions, including "How have you been wounded by the wrongs done to your ancestors?" (2008, p. 67). They also asked clients to explore how they have been affected by the wounds committed by their cultural group.

My colleague Natalie, besides being my Arizona road trip partner, teaches Multicultural Art Therapy with Diverse Populations at Southwestern College. I respect her passion regarding our students' understanding of who they are, who they come from, and what the lands are that they're from. She describes an intersectionality of information, a spiderweb of identity information that we received from our families. She emphasizes the idea of multiple identities.

In this context she requires that each student create a "Self-Geography Map" that reflects "personal ancestral identity, ancestral lands, immigration or rootedness, mixtures of 'culture, class, gender, ability, sexual orientation, aging, and geographical identities'" (Carlton, personal communication, May 9, 2014). Each project is then presented in class to peers and Natalie. My belief is that this open, spacious assignment in the first year of study, lays a vital foundation for the art-based genograms in our students' second year of study. Natalie and I have both been concerned at times, about the response of white students, who sometimes have held the stance that "We're all the same. We're all human," and therefore are dismissive of their own ethnic heritages. Natalie strongly feels that "White privilege allows one to say I don't have a culture. Whites can fade their ethnic heritage – when you're white you don't have to define yourself" (Carlton, personal communication, May 9, 2014). She shared stories of "dangerous unfolding" as they prod their family members for information. Many family stories are off-limits or are reluctantly revealed. Students report saying to their parents: "I don't know much about our family – why didn't you tell me about this before?" In my own therapy work with clients, I've been surprised at how many people of apparent European heritage say "We don't have a culture."

Sara is a student who really opened her heart to the process of finding out about her people, first through the self-geography map, and then with her art-based genograms. She resonated with Natalie's beliefs that learning the sense of place, the land where one's people lived, matters. Sara said that she always was enchanted by the hills of Kentucky, the part of the country that her father's family was from. She grew up in Ohio and was eager for trips to this other location of family. Her father, however, had a lingering sense of the shame of poverty that had been a big part of his childhood.

Sara spoke of her father's commitment to the Cherokee people and belief systems within his heritage. Sara's research showed that some family members were forced on the Trail of Tears, while some were able to escape and hide in the mountains. Sara describes her interest in her lineage becoming consuming as her family seemed split between the more known, larger family on her dad's side, the "have-nots," and the smaller more unknown Ohio family on her mother's side, the "haves." She would tackle a line of her family's history and trace it as far back as she could. "All of a sudden my sense of being connected to the world really started to feel real. I had a sense of belonging, an idea of how many lives had happened, the stories of the past becoming part of my story" (Patrick, personal communication, June 26, 2014). Judith Fein shared a similar feeling at the end of her book about her trip to her ancestral village:

> Suddenly, I felt as though there were people behind me, following me. I turned around, but no one was there. I continued walking. Again, I felt the presence of a lot of people in my wake. I spun around and was greeted by a chorus of voices. Although I didn't see anybody, I heard the Eastern European ancestors of many people like me calling out. 'Remember us. Don't forget us. Our story needs to be heard. Write our story. Write your story.' (2014, p. 233)

Sara shared that while connecting the dots, names of people, names of towns, emerged and pulled her into her history. At one point, looking at the mix of family in Kentucky, it became clear that "Part of my lineage had tried to kill off part of my lineage." Her interest and passion for family research flared up again with the art-based genogram project. She chose to create a mobile with all natural elements from the earth; wooden sticks and dried gourds (see Figure 9). She felt that the movement present would represent the metaphor of external forces, change, anything impacting the family.

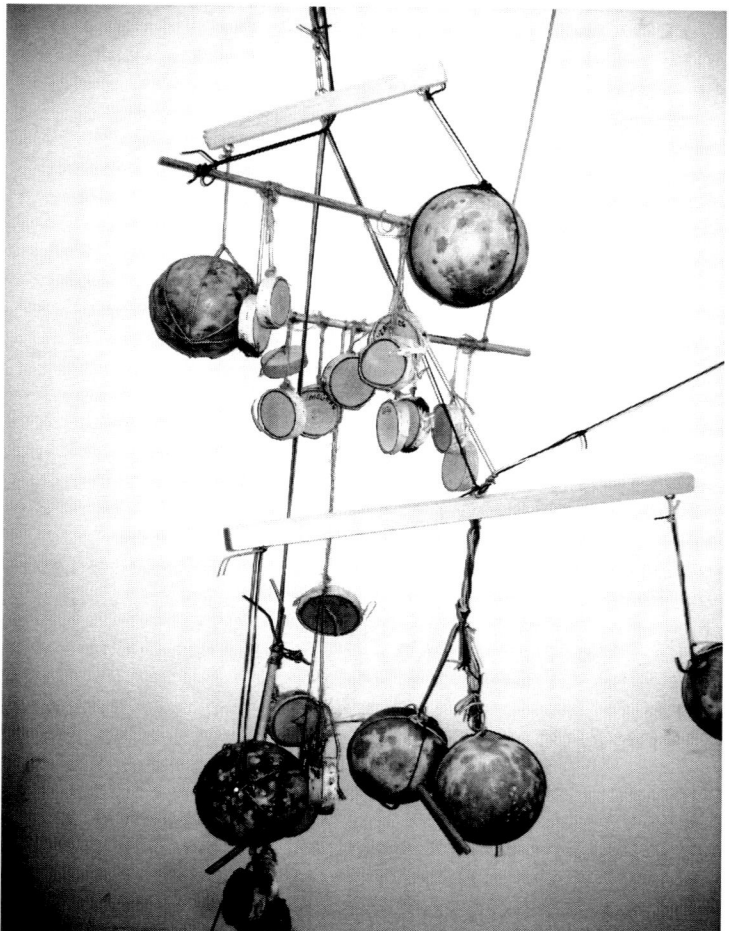

Figure 9. Genogram Mobile, Sara Patrick.

What resulted is one of the most honest art-based genograms that I've seen. It became a tangled mess. Sara said: "I couldn't get the pieces to stop moving. Things kept falling. I was trying to untangle the mess.

It became clear how each of us is affected in so many ways." She used the metaphor of the big knots: "I wanted to untangle the big knots so that people who come after me are free of these painful knots."

I asked Sara what the end result of all this hard work had been for her? "Forgiveness and compassion. Compassion keeps coming up for me. It's been powerful, it's moved me out of one story. My story is just one chapter in a really long family book (personal communication, June 26, 2014).

Knowing one's story is that vulnerable beginning place, I believe, in our paths to become people who offer healing to others. A native of Santa Fe, Val is a member of the Diné (Navajo) Nation, a "Two-Spirit" or transgender person, identifying as both male and female and so prefers the pronoun "they." They are also introverted and I appreciated their willingness to share their understanding of who they are, with me. I'd noticed the beautiful feather tattoo on Val's arm before, but I hadn't really seen it or their other tattoos up close (see Figure 10). Initially we met so that we could talk about a piece of art they had created that spoke to their cultural heritage and identities. The more we talked, the more I understood the depth of meaning of the imagery on their body. In addition to their Diné heritage, Val is half-white which accounts for the clipper ship tattooed near the feather on their arm. Val states: "we're from the colonized and the colonizer." Indigenous and immigrant, male and female, it seems appropriate that they described themselves as "a conduit with different energies running through, embodying a fluid concept of gender" (Jones, personal communication, July 17, 2014).

Val's solid understanding of who they are as Diné, Irish, Welsh, English, German, male and female, feels like a special treasure that when shared, widens my own appreciation for how we are human. Val spoke about feeling vulnerable, honest and open, when this sharing took place in the classroom among fellow art therapy students. Val found the experience of sharing to be healing, which continues to be an important aspect of knowing and sharing identities.

I believe that Val has the potential to offer much healing to others. Val has much to share and their understanding of multiple identities will bring a tender sensitivity to Val's future client work. I continue to be moved by all the beautiful spirits who move through our program and eventually share their healing gifts with the world.

Multicultural Gifts and Challenges Revealed

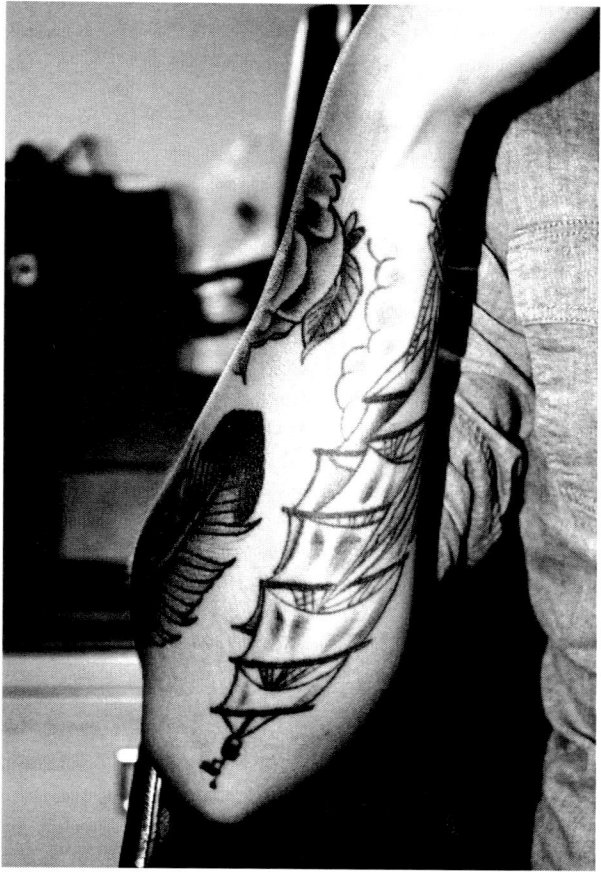

Figure 10. Tattoo, Val Jones.

While Val actually portrayed their heritage on their skin, another student, Laura, decided to create her artistic statement by sewing a dress containing her heritage that she could wear (see Figure 11). It was significant to Laura that it be wearable: "It's kind of a quilt with different stories." In order to create her dress, she needed to contact her grandma, who she is close to and she reported that speaking with her grandma about the family history was very touching: "She got really excited about this project, sharing information and stories with me."

The many patterns of fabric actually reminded me of the rows of crops that we see when we fly over farmland. Farming is an important theme in Laura's personal geography, and it shows up very early in family history. She can trace her family back to the very first farmers

84   *Exploring and Developing the Use of Art-Based Genograms*

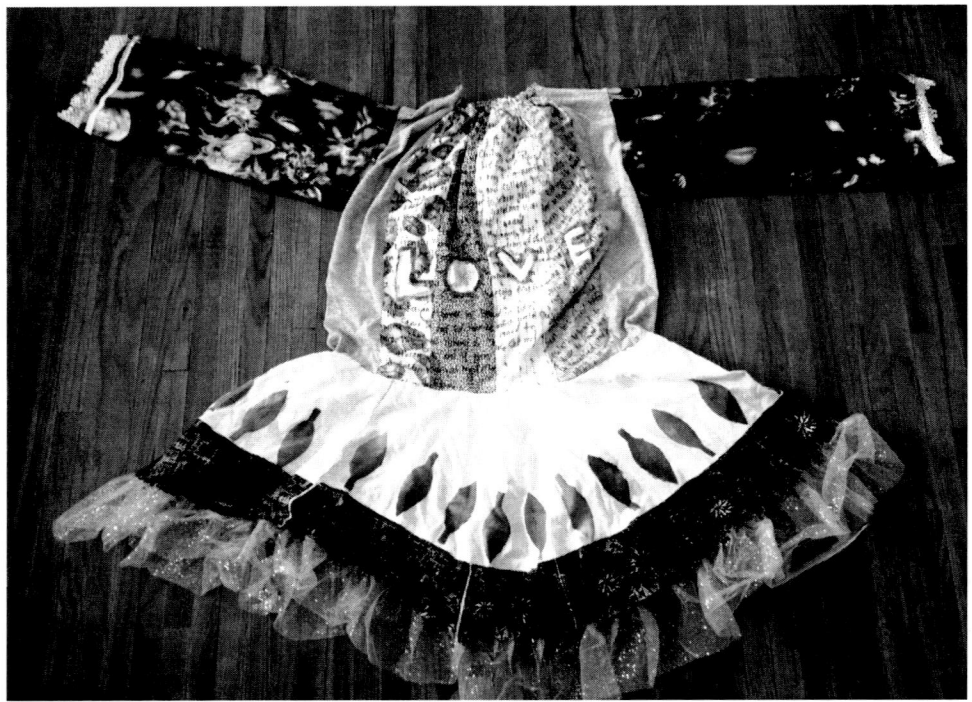

Figure 11. Dress, Laura Fischer.

who settled in Canada, bringing their ways of planting and harvesting with them from Europe.

Laura is an avid traveler and I wonder if perhaps her love of adventure is made possible because of her deeply grounded roots of "home." "I've always had a strong sense of home and place, and the dress project has contributed to that. Everywhere I've been, my family has stayed present for me" (Laura Fischer, personal communication, June 30, 2014).

I think that "home" can be a very wide word. What comes up for you when you hear that word? Is it the house or apartment where you live? Is it the place you were born or grew up in? Is it a geographical place that you most resonate with? Or is it the ancestral lands that your people came from? There is a luscious book titled *Personal Geographies: Explorations in Mixed-Media Mapmaking*, that Natalie discovered after she came up with her personal geographies assignment. Author Jill K. Berry stated: "I wanted to not only look at maps, but employ the act of making them into my art as a tool for storytelling and self-discovery"

(2011, p. 4). She offered ideas regarding three kinds of mapmaking – maps of physical self, maps of one's experience and "Dimensional projects with a cartographic theme. . . . In the end, you will have a personal atlas that is a visual memoir of your life" (p. 5).

And sometimes there is no need to create a memoir; sometimes people live in the places that have been imprinted on their hearts and souls since birth. People return to their places of birth, no matter how haunted those refuges are. The very walls recount the wounding. On an intimate, interpersonal level, sometimes I wonder how we can acknowledge cultural/racial wounding without moving into hopeless collapse. My partner Joey uses the symbol of his family's adobe home as a metaphor for the waves of struggle and trauma endured while growing up. His anger and exasperation surface when he talks about his continuous and seemingly futile attempts at repair and maintenance. Behind the metaphor is the reality of an old adobe home existing in a small village that has withstood invasions of hostile rivals from neighboring villages, hippies from the city, local heroin sellers and users, and tourists eager to own land in this beautiful setting.

And just under the surface of this history is the history of the Spanish conquest of indigenous Native land. The connections between families in northern New Mexico become painfully alive in stories of the north. My sorrow as witness to this pushes my ethical boundaries. I attempt to be some small encouraging voice toward healing while maintaining my role as partner, not therapist.

I feel encouraged by Gibson's words: "As painful as your story may be, it is the force in your life that propels you toward healing" (2008, p. 215). I like to imagine the rippling out of healing as it impacts children, grandchildren, and family members seven generations into the future (Gibson, 2008).

Chapter 13

THE INTERGENERATIONAL FLOW OF SPECIAL ISSUES

The presence of musical notes, tiny pianos, a saxophone and three violins, created a genogram that seemed like we could almost hear it while we looked at it. Georgia literally sang "We are family, I got all my sisters with me" while I tracked the visual melody of her family, present in her art-based genogram, through generations. I couldn't wait to understand the role that musical gifts played in her family's experience. This strength-based imagery was invited into the room to be present alongside a visual documentation about a number of early deaths relating to family members within her genogram.

Other clients have incorporated themes such as sports, types of employment, religion, creativity, recreational activities and pets into their genograms. It's intriguing to watch skills, interests and abilities flow across the generations. As you get to know your clients, you can listen for clues that can help amplify the strengths present but sometimes forgotten or not acknowledged with a client's history.

Anyone who's ever had a job that felt like torture can appreciate the need to bring employment-misery to therapy. We can help clients develop coping skills, work on stress reduction, look at career-fit, and other work-related issues. An art-based genogram can open up the conscious and unconscious family beliefs about levels of education, the "worthiness" of certain careers or jobs, and whether or not a type of employment "fits" with a family's view of itself in the world. I am reminded of Bowen's thoughts regarding the "togetherness factor." How often is a career choice a conscious or unconscious attempt at individuation?

A genogram that has a "work theme" can help clients explore some of the spoken and unspoken rules about work. Is it possible in a family of books (teachers) to decide to be a hammer (construction worker)? How do family members talk about people who are unemployed, underemployed, or doing work that is perceived as somehow "beneath" the family's work traditions? And conversely, there's also the "Who does she think she is?" factor that can be present when someone moves into an area of work that's thought of as being something that moves that person away from being "one of us."

Certainly the themes of health/medical concerns and mental health issues are focal points for many genograms. A predominance of any difficult condition, moving through several generations, can be frightening and the visual impact of seeing many greenish blobs, for example, representing cancer, can open up a place in our work together where fear and grief can be shared.

As I considered the variety of themes present in art-based genogram work, I remembered some visual references to eating disorders, when I asked families during the intensive family weekends at the residential treatment center, to create art-based genograms. In those particular families, though, the "identified client" often had an early trauma history which had set a variety of responses and issues into motion. During those fast family weekends, the focus was mostly on the traumas that had been experienced and the impact on family relationships.

I was curious about the existence of family of origin themes and issues present in work with eating disordered clients and so I contacted several art therapists who specialize in this area of work. A former student, art therapist Pat Lopez, has concentrated on working with clients at an eating disorder clinic. She provides group and individual art therapy and along with other therapists there, shares the evening meal with clients. I asked her to share any themes that she had experienced in terms of her clients' families of origin. She shared with me that "Food was not present as nourishment" (Lopez, personal communication, Nov. 21). It seems that food was anything but the sustaining fuel for her clients' bodies. Anita Johnston, Ph.D. spoke of some of the metaphors present in food and eating:

> For most of us, eating takes on meaning way beyond physical nutrition. It can be used as a substitute for love. . . . Eating can be used as a means of providing comfort and support at times when we are feeling sadness or pain. This is a relationship supported by many families

and by our culture. . . . Eating can be used to escape from uncomfortable feelings in much the same way that drugs and alcohol have been used and abused. (1996, p. 41)

Dr. Johnston also described how a child may learn to eat or not eat, as a stand against parents. In our conversation, Pat used a term that I had never heard of before; she asked if I remembered my first wounding with food? Pat said that her clients usually remembered the first time that they had an issue with food as happening between the ages of ten and thirteen. A sense of comparison seemed to become present for girls at that time. Not just to their mothers or sisters, but also to older brothers, other neighborhood kids, and as we know from story after story, images of women in the media. I think that most of us can identify the early messages that we received, good or bad, about who we were around the ages of ten to thirteen. It feels important, in an exploration of eating disorder origins, to explore the ideas of who we were in relationship to food and family.

Clinical psychologist and art therapist Lisa Hinz shared a number of art directives that she uses with clients, and I can envision several of them having a strong impact in family of origin work. She asked clients to: "Draw a picture of your family at the time the eating disorder started. Be sure to include each family member and draw your family engaged in an activity" (2006, p. 63). She also invited her client to include a number of contextual and cultural details of that time period. Visually, it must be fascinating to see how clients use color, shape, line, placement of family members, size, and prominence, to share the story of that time in family life.

> Discussing family dynamics helps patients determine what influences they were responding to as they were growing up. By examining the family drawing, patients will gain clues to parental discord, sibling rivalry, sibling physical or emotional illness, and other family influences that predisposed them to develop an eating disorder. (2006, p. 64)

Having asked many clients to create some type of family drawing, it makes sense to me to purposefully target the time when the disorder first presented. Even more intriguing to me is the directive that Hinz called "In my childhood kitchen" (p. 71). She asked clients to: "Imagine for a moment, what it was like to be in your childhood kitchen when a meal was being prepared. Remember what the kitchen looked like, what it smelled like, what it sounded like, and what it felt like. Remember some of the foods that you have tasted there" (p. 72).

Hinz also invited clients to indicate the presence of the person providing or making the food. Whether created with a realistic look or in abstract, this kind of image would seem to be filled with information, conscious memories, and unconscious impressions.

> In remembering their childhood kitchens, patients commonly report control of food, weight, and body image . . . they report having mothers who rigidly controlled what food was in the cupboard, when it was eaten, and by whom. These patients claim having little control over what they ate until the eating disorder developed . . . father who . . . curtailed their food choices, and vigilantly monitored their intake. Many report being placed on diet pills as early as elementary school ages. Frequently they report sneaking, hiding, and hoarding food in response to rigid control over their food intake and weight. (Hinz, 2006, p. 73)

In our conversation, Pat Lopez mentioned the mother-daughter relationship as often particularly powerful in terms of the context of the development of eating disorders. She spoke of the power that mothers had over daughters' choices. She also emphasized that her clients' mothers may or may not have actually had an eating disorder themselves. But they impacted their daughters' feelings about food, body image and changing/developing bodies in a myriad of ways (personal communication, Nov. 21, 2014).

Some mothers may experience envy toward their daughters' youthful, attractive bodies and become critical and competitive with them when they enter puberty and discover their sexuality. Compulsive eating or self-starvation may become a way for these daughters to distract themselves from feelings of confusion, estrangement, or anger (Johnston, 1996, p. 123).

When I reflect on the potential intersection of family rules about food and family rules about sex, I appreciate the skills that it takes in some families to navigate those early adolescent years. As bodies begin to change, the spoken and unspoken beliefs about eating, weight, sexuality and body image can be overwhelming.

Art therapist and marriage and family therapist Susan Perry Halvorson graciously shared some of her thoughts with me regarding her work with family of origin issues that have surfaced with her eating disorder clients:

When conducting an initial assessment with an eating disorder client, I take a thorough family history. More often than not the client has had or currently has a family member with an eating disorder. It is no surprise that genetic factors contribute to a predisposition for EDs and that EDs are heritable. It seems that individuals who are born with certain genotypes are at an increased risk for the development of an ED – for example, in my practice I often see personality traits such as obsessive thinking, perfectionism, emotional instability, impulsivity and rigidity passed down from a family member to a client.

Both spoken and unspoken rules play a factor in EDs being transmitted generationally. This can be an interesting art therapy directive. I often ask my ED clients to draw/write any unspoken or spoken rules that they have experienced in their family of origin related to food and body image. With spoken rules I often see everything from "eat everything on your plate" to "I wouldn't take a second helping if I were you. . . ." With unspoken rules, family members (most often a parent) model certain behaviors that become the "rule." One client drew a picture of her mother, her aunt and her grandmother all dressed the same in "perfect outfits." On each of their plates she drew a few small vegetables and salad. The men's plates had all the typical Thanksgiving fare. When talking about her picture, she said that all the women in her family were "thin and perfect and ate like birds." She believed that was expected of her as well. This particular client had been hospitalized for anorexia at 16 years old.

I often talk with clients about how our relationships with other people most influence our relationships with our own bodies. Starting in our families of origin and then moving to friends and significant others – all relationships shape our attitudes about our bodies. It seems true that no intimate relationship has more impact on our Body Image than the relationship we have with our mothers. Mothers that are present in their daughters' lives can have enormous influence over how a daughter perceives and relates to her own body and furthermore how she relates to food. It is no surprise that maternal eating disorders and childhood feeding problems go hand-in-hand.

The healing process from an ED is a long, arduous journey. If a client is still living with family members it is imperative that family therapy sessions are included in the treatment plan. Likewise, if the client is living with a spouse or significant other, it is important for him/her to be included in sessions from time to time. (Perry Halvorson, personal communication, Nov. 26, 2014)

Family members' abilities to be honest and open regarding their relationship to the client, their feelings about the eating disorder, and their willingness to look authentically at the impact of the client's actions and their own actions on one another would seem vital. Authors Richards, Hardman and Berrett shared a process similar to family sculpture experiences described in other chapters:

> The purpose of this intervention is for each family member to create "pictures," visually and spatially, of the patient's family, representing personal perceptions of the family and the place of the eating disorder in it. . . . This activity and period of sharing can lead to an open discussion on how the family could live together without the eating disorder as an unwanted "extra" family member. (2007, p. 153)

I am appreciative of the use of creativity and metaphor, in the treatment of this issue, that by its very nature, is metaphor for so many emotional and personal issues in human life. Another difficult issue that shares similar qualities with eating disorders, is the treatment of substance abuse.

A number of art therapy colleagues doing substance abuse work use genograms as they encourage clients to look at their families' histories with addictions. I remembered that Amy, former student of mine, had really made meaningful personal use of her own art-based genogram. I wasn't surprised to learn that she was asking clients in her therapy group (related to substance abuse issues) to create them: "The clients were able to get into the process using a variety of mediums and were able to make connections about their families and lineages. They liked the process of using art instead of doing a written-out family tree" (Vidra, personal communication, July 3, 2014).

Another art therapy colleague, Carrie, specialized for years working with addictions and underlying trauma. She shared:

> The genogram can be a powerful tool for creating awareness in individuals struggling with addictions. When used properly it can inspire an "aha" experience for clients who are connecting the dots of how and when they learned to cope by using addictive thinking and behavior to numb feelings.
>
> It is essential that all types of addictive behaviors be included on the genogram including substances, processes, and codependent behaviors. Too often assessments are focused exclusively on substance use while many other types of addictive behaviors go undetected. This can lead to scapegoating the "addict" whose behavior is most out

of control, and can prevent opportunities for greater awareness and healing within the larger family system.

Substance abuse can include drugs, alcohol, cigarettes, and caffeine. Process addictions can include shopping, hoarding, gambling, internet, and sex addictions. Eating disorders should also be included on the genogram as they often coexist with substance abuse and have their own unique pattern of distorted thinking.

Whereas it is very helpful for an individual to uncover the familial roots of his or her style of coping, full recovery is dependent upon the addict taking full responsibility for his or her behavior. The genogram is not meant as a vehicle for blaming the family system, but as an instrument of consciousness. Recovery includes the healing of underlying emotional wounds, learning to experience feelings rather than to numb them, and making amends to others they have harmed while "using." (Ishee, personal communication, July 1, 2014)

Georgia, my client with the musical genogram, also included many tiny alcohol bottles in her art. She was able to share that she'd been drinking pretty heavily following the recent sudden death of a nephew. We cried together over the violent end to such a young life. While noticing the many symbols for alcohol next to so many images of family members, she decided that she was willing to look at some other ways to sit with her grief.

Grief and loss issues can sit side-by-side with happy memories, in the art-based genograms of children who have lived with multiple families. I've helped kids create these precious maps using art, in order to preserve their own histories. Danny was in the process of connecting with a solid adoptive family, after four different other families. His biological parents hadn't been able to sustain any kind of reasonable care for him, and he'd gone to live with a grandma whose health failed and couldn't take care of him. Next, a foster family where an older kid beat him up. The sad litany of "family" seemed ready to dramatically change as his current family was kind and good and nurturing, and most importantly, wanted to have him with them forever.

Danny was happy and scared at the same time. He verbally repeated his story of people, over and over, and it felt to me as though he was repeating it in order to save it. Consequently we did save it, with art, mapping out symbols for everyone, writing names and dates beside the symbols, documenting seven years of family. "We believe that genograms can be a particularly useful tool for tracking children in multiple contexts. The many different family constellations children may live in are otherwise extremely hard to keep in mind. The more clear clinicians are in tracking this history, however complex, the better able to validate the child's actual experience and multiple forms of belonging" (McGoldrick, Gerson, & Petry, 2008, p. 153). We made a special art folder to keep his art-based family story in, and I made a copy for his new family, and a copy for my records. His people, his experiences, and his memories mattered, and they provided a launching place for the next important chapter of family for him.

Chapter 14

TOXIC GREEN CHALK

Ripped up before a photo could be taken, I can only describe what I remember about Rita's art-based genogram. She started with black paper as a background and then drew small brown doors to represent most of her family. Although people joke about "skeletons in the closet," these skeleton-filled closets were drawn with serious determination. She began speaking as she worked, telling the family secrets that an elderly aunt had finally shared with her. Rita described an unwanted pregnancy hidden behind one door, several generations in the past, that had ended with the baby being raised as the young mother's "sister" and the young mother's eventual suicide. The baby eventually grew into a "wild woman" with numerous stories of multiple partners attached to her name. Eventually she married and gave birth to Rita's mother who could only be described as puritanical. As teenagers, Rita and her sister had joked about how in the world they could have come into existence, given their mother's apparent stance on sex.

"We didn't know any of this, but I think we knew it deep down, inside. There were secrets everywhere and we knew better than to ask about any family members. We lived far away from everyone and all the secrets." It would seem that moving away from other family members had probably helped her mother maintain the deep secrets. Rita continued: "We couldn't ever figure out what was wrong, but we knew something was." Not being able to understand unspoken family rules and not even being able to ask any questions, can make children feel crazy. "When parents keep their feelings a secret, their children often become confused and anxious. . . . Genetic predispositions often coincide with family dynamics, and a child may take on unresolved feelings of sadness that have come from previous generations" (Bradshaw, 1995, p. 49). Bradshaw continues, describing this experience as the "felt sense" (p. 49) of the family. Rita could describe carrying a sense that something was wrong, but not having any words about it.

Rita sat in silence for a while with her rows of closed closet doors. Slowly she began encircling the topmost row of doors with a neon-green chalk pastel. She ran her fingers over it, adding more chalk, then began smearing the green down to the next level of family, and the next. She called it the "toxic slime" of the family, and eventually it was smeared over her own self-image which was a bird in a cage. I couldn't help but be aware of my own inner yearning for the bird to fly out of the cage before it was suffocated by the green slime. (As a way to process the session after Rita left, I created an image of her bird flying free.) Rita continued rubbing the green chalk into the black paper, crying as her finger broke through the paper and made a hole. She pushed back her chair and grabbed the paper, ripping it up, leaving a metaphoric pile of sadness on the table.

Rita had come to therapy because she wanted to make her marriage work. She knew her husband of four years was frustrated with her and she was frustrated, too. "He says I don't seem real sometimes. I don't always know what's real inside; I don't know what I'm feeling so I put on a happy face. "Often genuine feelings are not available – due to defenses or repression or denial. When we meet shame, we recognize that we often are meeting the masking of affect, and realize that we need to get behind the mask to find the person" (Fossum & Mason, 1986, p. 37). This disconnect from her own feelings, her own self, in order to protect ancestors unknown secrets was taxing her ability to show up authentically in an intimate relationship. "Toxic shame affects not just our *doing* but our very *being*. . . . Toxic shame demands that I wear a mask, put on a disguise, develop a false self. If I were to let you see me as I really am, you would see that I am flawed and defective and reject me" (Bradshaw, 1995, p. 30).

To make matters worse, Rita had grown up in an atmosphere of tight control and had taken that in as her way of being in the world. Bradshaw named control as the first in his list of "The Dysfunctional Family Rules" (1998, p. 39). The list begins with (1). Control – One must be in control of all interactions, feelings and personal behavior at all times . . . control is the major defense strategy for shame" (IBID). Rita used control to feel safe. It might not seem logical but sticking to her schedule, keeping the apartment spotless, and knowing where her husband was at all times, were ways to keep the anxiety of the unknown at bay. "Commonly, the control principle is motivated not so much by a drive to power as by a drive for predictability and safety" (Fossum & Mason, 1986, p. 88). There was therefore, no room for flexibility or spontaneity in Rita's marriage, creating a cage not only for herself, but also for her husband.

Over time, Rita made some peace with her family's history. She eventually created a kind of simple shrine to the young mother who died, and the baby, and her own mother's protection of what she must have understood as a terribly shameful legacy. She kept the shrine in my office closet which I think was a kind of metaphoric protection from letting the shrine enter her home. Some of the issues that were held so tightly by previous generations can puzzle us now. More than a few clients have told me about divorces that were held as unacceptable secrets, only being spoken of at funerals. And many, many clients shared that their conception happened before their parents were married, which in some families continues to be held as a serious family secret.

And some secrets were understandably shut away in closets, not ever included in any version of the family narrative, but still felt and sensed by family members and persistently shared generationally. Bradshaw wrote of using the genogram as "the primary tool in deciphering my family secrets" (1995, p. 100). He stated: "When I drew my own genogram, I was surprised to find some startling similarities over the three generations. . . . I found some dark secrets that had directly impacted my life and impaired my freedom. I had been acting out things that were never talked about" (IBID).

It intrigues me that the knowledge that there is some kind of dark family secret is transmitted, but the overt knowledge of the secret itself can remain unknown. The family creates a way of being in the world that maintains and protects itself. "Unconscious mutual contracts of inattention between a husband and wife are extended to the children. All the members of the family unconsciously agree to a number of shared blind spots or secrets that govern what can be noticed and talked about and what is not to be noticed or spoken about" (Bradshaw, 1995, p. 75).

Often something happens that brings a member of the family into therapy and the therapist may get the sense that there's more going on than the stated problem. And so we build relationship and gently hold the space for safety and containment and then the underlying secret tentatively enters the room, in my experience most often through the art. The client who seems dysthymic creates a dark hole of despair and together we explore what's in there. Sexual abuse? Emotional abuse? Generations of financial failure?

My first visit to a therapist was to stop the debilitating panic attacks that I was having. New to therapy, I didn't understand the wider context for what we talked about in session. Looking back I believe that I unconsciously shared my anxious way of being in the world with my two young sons. Parenting from a core of fear looks and sounds different from parenting from an inner sense of safety and trust. "Repressed emotions often feel too big, like they would completely overwhelm us if we expressed them. There is also the fear of the shame that would be triggered if we expressed our emotions" (Bradshaw, 1988, p. 55).

Researchers have had some fascinating results when exploring the transgenerational transmission of fear, using mice. Using "olfactory molecule specificity," Dias and Ressler conditioned mice to fear a particular odor prior to conception (Dias & Ressler, 2013). The next two generations of mice exhibited behavioral sensitivity to the odor that the parent mice had been conditioned to be afraid of. The benefits, generationally, are clear – the next generations of mice were warned about something that they might encounter in their environment someday. It was found that the experiences of the parent before conceiving the offspring influenced both the structure and function in the nervous system of subsequent generations. "Such a phenomenon may contribute to the etiology and potential intergenerational transmission of neuropsychiatric disorders, such as phobias, anxiety and posttraumatic stress disorder" (Dias & Ressler, 2013, p. 95).

It feels promising to me, that even though the experiment was with mice, it seems to be validating that felt sense, or instinctual response that we humans experience on an unconscious level in the spots we hold in our families' histories. Any conscious attempt to learn the intergenerational transmission of fear, sadness or shame would seem to be a precious gift to the next generation.

Chapter 15

WIDENING OUR VIEWS, WORKING WITH COLLEAGUES

Sometimes being a therapist can feel a little isolative, especially in private practice because one can yearn for the support and warmth of colleagues, which can be a lovely part of agency life. In Wisconsin I looked forward to our weekly treatment team meetings because the women on those intensive in-home teams were so much fun to work with. In the absence of a whole team of smart, caring, funny therapists, I've managed to be very lucky in terms of cofacilitation opportunities with other professionals. I like the creative zing that collaborative work offers.

A few years ago, Kate Cook, a relationally-oriented expressive therapist and trainer, invited me to cofacilitate a workshop with her, and I appreciated this opportunity to come to know more about how she works. She uses psychodrama, sand tray, and action methods along with other expressive approaches, and so I was interested in her thoughts about incorporating these creative methods in family of origin work. Kate grounds her expressive therapy work in interpersonal neurobiology.

Siegel's work has long helped us to understand the vital importance of this foundation that Kate works from. He spoke of the brain as a living system, "an integrated collection of component subsystems that interact together. . . . A living system that must be open to the influences of the environment in order to survive" (Siegel, 1999, p. 16). He continued, speaking of the system of a brain becoming "functionally linked to other systems, especially to other brains" (p. 17). These other brains are the humans surrounding a person and so it is no surprise that as knowledge about how the brain works seems to multiply daily, the field of infant mental health has exploded in terms of importance.

These connections between brains involve what he describes as resonance "in which energy and information are free to flow" between brains and "when interpersonal communication is 'fully engaged' – when the joining of minds is in full force – there is an overwhelming sense of immediacy, clarity, and authenticity" (Siegel, 1999, p. 337). A therapist working from a strong base of interpersonal neurobiology would necessarily understand the power of relationships within a family (and of course also outside the family) to enable healing to happen.

From her therapeutic work, Kate states: "In family of origin work people can give a left-hemisphere verbal narrative, but when you ask them to put it into metaphor or imagery, what is transmitted is the spirit of the family. So much more depth, texture and detail is shared. Relationships are more accurately depicted" (Cook, personal communication, June 25, 2014). Kate often asks a family to move from imagery to action; after they create an art statement, she asks them to enliven it, bring it into motion, let it speak. "Rhythm, metaphor, movement, dance, are the language of the right brain."

Kate has frequently cofacilitated trainings with Bonnie Badenoch. Both clinicians use their knowledge of attachment theory and interpersonal neurobiology as core elements in family of origin work. Bonnie spoke to the issue of family histories in her book *Being a Brain-wise Therapist: A Practical Guide to Interpersonal Neurobiology:* "Listening to history can be less about learning the facts and more about thoroughly dropping into the world of the other" (2008, p. 163). She spoke about using the genogram format and states:

> It will be helpful to ask for history about at least three generations . . . this longitudinal approach can build the foundation for *intergenerational compassion.* . . . As we listen and begin to understand the warmth and resources that have been passed down in the family, our empathy for each member will touch our patient, even if it happens initially below the level of consciousness. (p. 164)

I've long been intrigued by the *Inner Community* work that Bonnie writes about. Based in object relations theory, attachment theory and interpersonal neurobiology, the paradigm is formed around "the centrality of relational experience in shaping the inner world" (2008, p. 77). She continued: "Inner community focuses on the way we take in, and then live out, the relationships we internalize in both our earliest days and throughout life" (p. 78). I know that my own inner community includes everyone within my genogram, plus a wide array of people and characters who impacted me over the years. I was an avid reader as a young girl and I feel like some of those significant literary relationships helped shape who I am in the world. I played a little one day with a kind of literary genogram and girls and women from a variety of books showed up in my art. Laura from the *Little House on the Prairie* series was there, hanging out with *Mara, Daughter of the Nile*, and several of the sisters from *Little Women*.

When clients have moved through life with a significant absence of a biological parent, I often ask where they got some mothering or fathering from, and if they have children, where they learned how to be a mom or a dad. I'm not surprised when clients have been favorably impacted by well-loved characters in books and films. Similar in some ways to the idea of inner communities, is the work of Richard Schwartz in his *Internal Family Systems Model*. He presented the concept that we think about our relationships to our own thoughts and emotions in a new way, and that healing can evolve through building new relationships with all of those "parts" (2001). I think that we all organically speak about our "parts" at times. "In other words, it is as if we each contain a society of people, each of whom is at a different age and has different interests, talents, and temperaments" (Schwartz, 1995, p. 34). I certainly am aware of an "Anxious Debbie" who seems to rely on the appearance of who I call my "Inner Extrovert." It takes a lot of energy for me to summon the extroverted part and I think it might be fun to create images of these parts, someday. I suspect that they may resemble some of the images that appear in my art-based genogram.

I was delighted to come across the work of Somatic Art Therapist, Somatic Experiencing Practitioner, and Internal Family Systems Therapist, Dr. Meagan Pugh, at an American Art Therapy Association Conference. I contacted her and she generously agreed to speak with me about her work which combines art therapy, somatic experiencing and Internal Family Systems. She has done what she referred to as "parts work" for most of her art therapy career. She emphasized the importance of therapists doing their own work and spoke about imaging parts of herself and dialoging with them, a process that echoes shamanic traditions of recalling lost energies, archetypes. She shared this about her work:

> The Internal Family Systems model helps clients heal by building compassionate relationships with the emotional, physical, spiritual and mental coping strategies they developed as a result of early life experience. These sensations, feelings and thoughts are called parts or inner cast of characters.
>
> Some of those inner parts are staunch protectors and managers that are developed to protect from future threat. A few of these protective parts are tyrannical in their attempts to keep the inner system from overwhelm and continue to operate as if a person is still young and helpless. Known as the Critic, Controller, Inner Perpetrator, Dissociater and Pusher, these coping strategies are relentless and addictive. In the language of IFS, they 'drive the bus.'
>
> With somatic awareness practices, creative art processes and the Internal Family Systems model, one can identify and transform these behaviors from tyrants into helpful allies. This supports the nervous system to release the aftereffects of early trauma and bring the overall system into calmness and clarity. (Pugh, personal communication, Nov. 15, 2014)

Working from a nonpathological stance, she spoke of "the parts" as having agendas to protect, and at one time, being great resources for an individual. She invites people to create images or three-dimensional representations of a part as it naturally surfaces in therapy. She used the example of someone saying "I have a knot in my stomach." Meagan would then invite them to create the knot, using art. Is the knot heavy? Is it rough? Once the art has been created, the client can respond to it. She calls taking the inside feeling and putting it outside, "making a hard copy." Once it's outside, her clients realize that they are indeed bigger than the image. They can feel empowered to be curious about it and eventually even move into compassion for the origination and role that the part has played in the client's life. And then, just as in the other art processes described in prior chapters, the idea of choice appears.

Meagan spoke of parts being stuck in their rather rigid roles and how the art process can "unblend" them. She spoke about the shifts that can happen and how she views her work as being a cotherapist with her clients, empowering them to go within. This is reflected in her statement "I know from an embodied place, as humans we have the capacity to heal ourselves" (Pugh, personal communication, Nov. 15, 2014). I appreciate the way that Meagan listens for those moments in conversation with a client when metaphor is present in words and then can move into being present in art. This is a style of work and a way of deepening the conversation with a client that seems to flow organically.

I think that one of the issues that new therapists struggle with is interviewing and obtaining information in a manner that feels congruent with their own interpersonal style and that feels comfortable for the client. I remember a number of students over the years who were horrified at the sound of these interviews when we listened to recordings of their session. "I sound like I'm interrogating him!" My hope is that art therapists remember to use art in this process!

My colleague Ani who is a marriage and family therapist and cofacilitated family therapy with me, appreciated the power of the art: "It brought a way of introducing information, and not forcing it out of the clients" (Tiffany, personal communication, June 11, 2014). My own belief that the art that needs to show up today, *will* show up today, helps me relax a little in the information-gathering process. As we externalize the issue or problem, using art, it usually feels more possible for the client to sit with it. Externalization is a powerful force in therapeutic work, and I invited my friend Carolyn, a verbal therapist, to speak about her use of metaphor in family of origin work:

> Trained in narrative therapy techniques, I have long used techniques that help externalize the problem. Instead of focusing on concepts such as you are an angry person, I focus on the externalized anger entering a relationship or situation. And so when anger enters, what happens? How can we reduce the power of anger when it decides to enter? Similarly, we can then look at the stories clients choose to tell and the language they use.
>
> In narrative therapy, as with many cognitive models, the identifying of the patterns is partly an uncovering of the stories we choose to tell ourselves about ourselves and our own histories and our worlds. The idea is to look with curiosity at how we've developed our personas, our ways of navigating the world, and to explore in what ways we may want to shift those patterns, personas, ways of being, if the patterns themselves, developed as protections, have now become problems.
>
> Sometimes with individuals or families I use the genogram to explore together the patterns that have developed within families. I use a fairly large piece of paper, and we take our time – sometimes a few sessions, or parts of sessions, to see the patterns emerge. . . . I use the regular symbols – circles for women, squares for men, and then I ask the client to choose three words that they feel most accurately de-

scribe the kind of person they are; people choose words like kind, or stubborn, or creative, or odd duck, or anxious, or thoughtful. We look at those words together — I hear stories regarding how they embody those words in their lives and relationships, and then we look at the underside of those words. What is the underside of being a helper, for example? If there is more than one person present, I ask permission for everyone to speak their experiences of these descriptions. Yes, someone might say, mom is a helper but sometimes she gets resentful and I can't seem to say no and things get weird. As we add other family members to the genogram . . . and look at descriptive words and how they resonate with each other, I can see clients becoming fascinated and more and more curious.

What is interesting is that the genogram can then truly be a non-threatening tool for just seeing what is, without taking on judgment and shame about what is. To externalize characteristics of people like this does not feel threatening to most people, and can give a sense that it might not be so impossible to shift even just a little, one's automatic responses. (Erickson, personal communication, July 15, 2014)

Clinical psychologist and author Louis Cozolino confirmed the value of stories, and oral storytelling as important factors in how we understand our experiences and our place in the family or world. "Memories are not a file of notes; they are stories that are told, reorganized, and recreated with each telling. Each time a memory is accessed, it can be modified (both in its narrative and neurology) by new experiences" (2006, p. 334).

My own therapeutic work has been enhanced and brightened by working with, talking with, and laughing with my colleagues. I think that in terms of scope of practice, we want to be aware that we can only offer to clients what we've been appropriately trained in, and I think that some of my best growth as a therapist has happened from listening to how my colleagues work, and then deeply examining my own therapeutic stance and skills. We never stop learning in this work.

I've always preferred the metaphor of a tossed salad to the "melting pot" image. In a tossed salad each element stays true to its unique flavor. No element really turns into something else. I encourage clinicians to be lively ingredients in the therapy salad, retaining their own unique views and gifts, while bumping up against ideas that add new colors and spice to the bowl.

Chapter 16

RETURNING, FINDING MEANING

Wendy has a smile that can light up a room. She was glowing when she came into my office and said "I'm redoing my genogram!" I was surprised. It's not unusual for difficult artwork to be destroyed and I seemed to remember that her art-based genogram had landed in the dumpster. As it turned out, the subsequent versions haven't felt satisfactory, either, to Wendy, and the new, improved version doesn't exist yet. Wendy's urge to revisit the creation of her genogram is completely understandable. Her first one was very dark, very gray. Wendy remembered: "I had a really hard time finding a way to be creative with it. I started to get really depressed with the imagery. I'd printed out black and white pictures and placed them on gray paper. The gray represented my family's depressing past." The gray clearly was appropriate as Wendy's story unfolded.

Using a tree theme, every branch of this art-based genogram held something really tough to talk about. Certainly the darkest memory was the point where her maternal grandfather escaped the Holocaust yet lost everyone else in his entire family. Wendy said that her grandfather could never talk about it. When her grandmother died, Wendy's mom was only thirteen and left with her father who relied on her for everything.

Wendy's mom had a sister who eventually entered into an abusive relationship and when Wendy's mom tried to intervene on behalf of her sister and later, her nieces, Wendy's grandfather put a dramatic stop to it saying "You don't break up a family!" This was a poignant response from someone whose family had been destroyed. Unfortunately, Wendy's mom continues to be blamed for not stepping in and rescuing her nieces.

The paternal side of Wendy's genogram was no happier, and as the whole art statement grew "It didn't get better." There were images related to premature death, divorce, abandonment, loneliness and possible sexual abuse. There were only very tiny slices of color that indicated fleeting glimpses of happiness. The genogram seemed to overflow with smart, accomplished people, but kindness and joy were clearly lacking.

I asked Wendy to talk a little about why she wanted to face this sad history again. "I felt the need to do it in a way that's more beautiful. I needed to visually shift it. I wanted a representation that's more aesthetically pleasing . . . and . . . it still looks ugly to me. I want it to look nice, to look pretty." I am moved by this honesty. How does one sit with bleak sadness and not move into despair? Even as Wendy grieves the idea that the family's Jewish traditions are disappearing, her hope for the future is based on love. She's been watching old home videos and capturing stills that hold tiny moments of happiness when she stops and freezes the frame. She laughs when I ask her how she does it: "What's the alternative? I have a choice to make and I choose to laugh. The genogram made me more aware of the darkness within my family history but it doesn't define me" (Wasserman, personal communication, May 28, 2014).

Gabor Maté (2009), in his book *In the Realm of Hungry Ghosts* wrote:

> Compassionate curiosity directed toward the self leads to the truth of things. . . . It is clear to me that the sense of threat and fear of abandonment that make up anxiety were, in my case, programmed in the Budapest ghetto in 1944. Why attempt to escape some old brain pattern laid down when I was a frightened infant during a terrible time in history? . . . The circuits in which its wordless stories are embedded are indelibly a part of my brain. It doesn't need to go away . . . but I can transform my relationship to it. (p. 357)

"Compassionate curiosity" is a wonderful phrase, although I can't help but think of those whose curiosity about biological family may never be satisfied.

Katherine shared her art and story with me. A vibrant young woman with a loving adoptive family, she wasn't sure how to look at the idea of who she is in the context of family. She was in Natalie's multicultural class and was asked to create her "Personal Geography." Katherine shared "It forced me to define myself. There was nothing really definitive based on my birth. I didn't look at what adoption meant to me until this assignment. I wondered, if you don't know, is there really a loss? When I thought about how this assignment applied to me I decided to explore how I've shaped who I am" (Monroe, personal communication, May 15, 2014). Joe Soll wrote: "An adoptee's existential experience is totally different from that of a non-adoptee. Therefore, the therapist often has no idea of and cannot imagine what her client's inner world even looks like" (2000, p. 115).

Her art exploration involved painting symbols from her life history on rocks and stacking them, creating a sculpture of what has defined her as a woman and as a person in relationships (see Figure 12).

> For the adoptee, it is as if she is an actress who has been dropped into the middle of the wrong movie. What is her real role? Who is she supposed to be.... She has to figure out what to do from now on, without knowing what happened in the past. In many ways she has no foundation to build on and she may develop a real fear of making mistakes in her life. (Soll, 2000, p. 86)

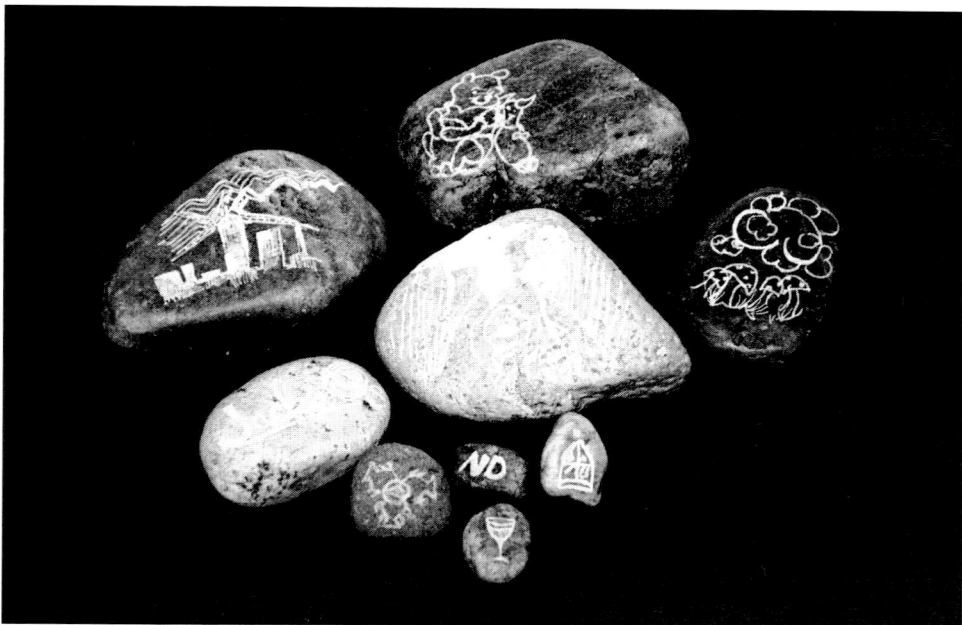

Figure 12. Rocks, Katherine Monroe.

As I listened to Katherine and examined her painted rocks, I thought about my daughter who is adopted. Katherine's rocks inexplicably wouldn't stack up neatly the day she shared them with me. Kind of an interesting metaphor, I think. I have to wonder what my daughter would define as key elements in her own development. I forget sometimes that I can't possibly understand her experience because my experience of our relationship is impossibly obscured by my love for her.

I have no doubt that Katherine will add more rocks to her art statement as life experiences and growing inner wisdom continue to shape and grow her definition of self. Perhaps the sculpture is simply waiting for that next rock to help it balance again. I like the idea that not only can my art grow and change over time, but so can my response to it. I appreciate the depth of meaning that is available when we live with our art and keep meaningful pieces accessible to us. Teri shared how her art-based genogram and its accompanying altered book have continued to impact her:

> Three years have passed since I did the genogram that emerged from a dream about dirt. Who would have thought that a simple dream would lead to such a healing and renewal. The dream led me to create a nontraditional genogram which depicted garden imagery with brightly colored flowers and garden dwellers such as frogs, birds, lizards and more. The fertile soil produced weeds and flowers alike. There was a theme of tremendous growth and abundance. Everything and anything could emerge from such a garden! Although many aspects of the genogram felt celebratory, there was plenty of sober reflection as well. I recognized some challenges we as a family faced, and could acknowledge the skeletons in the closet as our weeds in the garden This is what I recall these years later.
>
> The altered book I created as an additional process to the genogram has been on a table at home in easy reach. I thumb through the rough cardboard pages whenever the spirit moves me. As I look at the imagery I feel deep gratitude for my dream and all that it has birthed. I return to the dream again and again breathing in the rich smell of the fertile soil and affirming the thousands of years of family that led to my being here today.
>
> As I review the pages, I feel a vibrancy and healing presence resides there. It is as though this simple art book has morphed into a wonderful source of beauty, comfort, and celebration for me. The pages where I explore gold from the mother line and from the father line are especially meaningful. I am able to visually see the prosperi-

ty brought to me by my ancestors – spirituality, humor, music, ambition, hard work, creativity and more. It is a great source of comfort and affirmation for me.

I know that over these many years as an adult, there has been quite a bit of attention paid to wounds from family of origin issues. I have journal exploring, reviewing and working through one issue or another. I do not regret any of it. I am so glad, however, for the opportunity to blossom into a new and more affirming perspective of my family and myself. It, frankly, is a more balanced and honest representation of my family.

I shared my creative genogram with my mother and one of my brothers and they both enjoyed it. My mother, in particular, found the creations to be wonderfully affirming for her in her own journey. She became excited as she turned the pages of the altered book and saw our history – the good as well as the not so good. To this day, she will still mention the altered book and what its creation meant to her. I think it actually brought some peace to her which is something I had not anticipated.

The art-based genogram has provided me and family members with a deeper experience of the family soul and greater potential for healing. It is a process that I would recommend to others, and one I would certainly use as a therapist with my clients. (Teri, personal communication, 2014).

This acknowledgment that Teri has deeply experienced this process before she asks clients to do it, feels critical to me. The sense of oneself with a solid, knowing core of one's history is exactly what I hope that students and therapists gain from creating their own art first.

Nancy, a first-year student in Natalie's class, shared her experience and art (see Figure 13) with me:

The family geography art project I did for my Multicultural Diversity class was the hardest and yet most honest work I have ever done. . . . When I finished, I just stared at it. There were several feelings that sat with me. Fear. I was absolutely petrified that I was being so open about my life, my family and things that happened to me that I never talked about. Sick. I felt physically nauseous about what I had done, that I was going to present this piece. Pride. I did feel a sense of relief about the work I just finished. I was proud that I was taking this step. For me, I never really talk much; I am not good at expressing myself. The art piece I made was a miracle for me.

The project had a huge impact on me. It brought about a confidence in me I never really felt before. I feel more comfortable talking

110   *Exploring and Developing the Use of Art-Based Genograms*

about my life and my feelings when I am asked. This was partly due to my classmates who were very caring and accepting of my project and presentation.... Lastly, the healing power of art has impacted me the most. What I have trouble expressing in words, art has helped with this. Art has helped me open up. I know, after this art project I made, that I am on the right path in studying to be an art therapist. . . . This project was in many ways, life changing for me. I am grateful for the opportunity to make it. (Lemmon, personal communication, July 10, 2014)

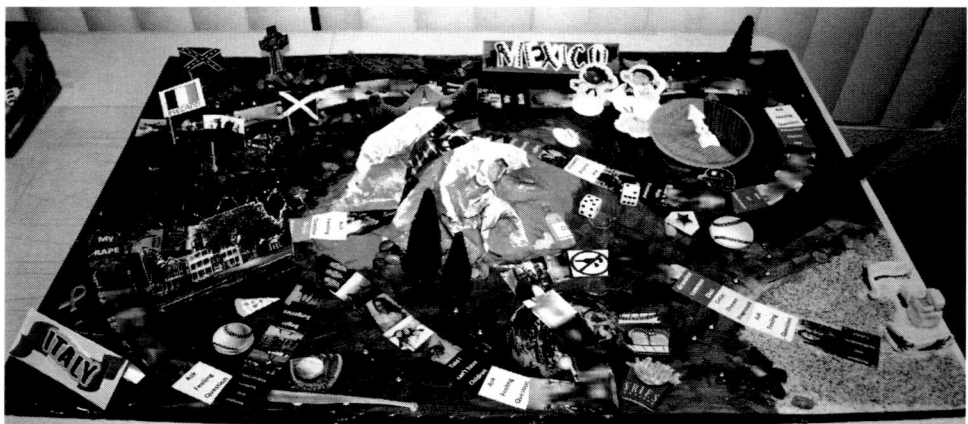

Figure 13. Game, Nancy Lemmon.

I also am grateful for the strength of anyone willing to do this often difficult exploration and sharing of family stories. No matter how the stories become visible in the art, (even the tragic stories, even the symbols of trauma), once they are visible, we have choice. We can choose whether the volcano's way of being, or the dolphin's way of interacting in the world, are embraced and then bestowed upon the next generation.

As I kiss my grandsons' warm faces I am creating my own place with each of them, in their own family histories. I feel a soft, bright sense of hope; I feel the power and responsibility to impact my own family in a way that nurtures joy and health. I am unabashedly that optimistic for each human and the far-reaching potential of any interaction that moves out to touch other humans with love.

EPILOGUE

CONNECTING THE DOTS

I was adding the finishing touches to this book when Wendy stopped by. Her eyes seemed to sparkle with a secret light and I was eager to find out why. I didn't have to ask, her words tumbled out quickly: "I was able to re-do my genogram, and I like it. I feel good about it!" Excited to see the new version, I asked her to bring it in. I was stunned when I saw it (see Figure 14). Created with natural materials and shimmering with a touch of gold paint, it's beautiful. When Wendy spoke about creating it, I knew I wanted to close this book with her story.

Her original art-based genogram had landed in the dumpster. Now, she and I both wish that she'd kept it, just to experience the contrast between the two art statements. This new genogram is a mobile and Wendy explained that "it needed to have two sides, my family has two sides and isn't two-dimensional." Crafted out of cardboard, rough rope, images of earth-toned textures and wire, its presence and feeling of nature reflects for Wendy, the idea that she's come to a more peaceful place with her family and family history. When she tried to re-do her genogram the first time, she said that she "couldn't see past the gray and black of the original one." She "couldn't see the colors."

As we looked at the genogram together, Wendy pointed out that it wasn't perfect – there are places that won't hang perfectly. Wendy reflected: "I was so tempted to make it perfect. But I had to let it be. You can't fix everything." A statement that truly speaks to family dynamics, it also acknowledges that the sadness present in her family history cannot be changed. Wendy spoke about the delicacy of the thin, fragile wire that holds the genogram together. A deep appreciation for the fragility of our time together in relationships on this planet is present in this art piece.

112 *Exploring and Developing the Use of Art-Based Genograms*

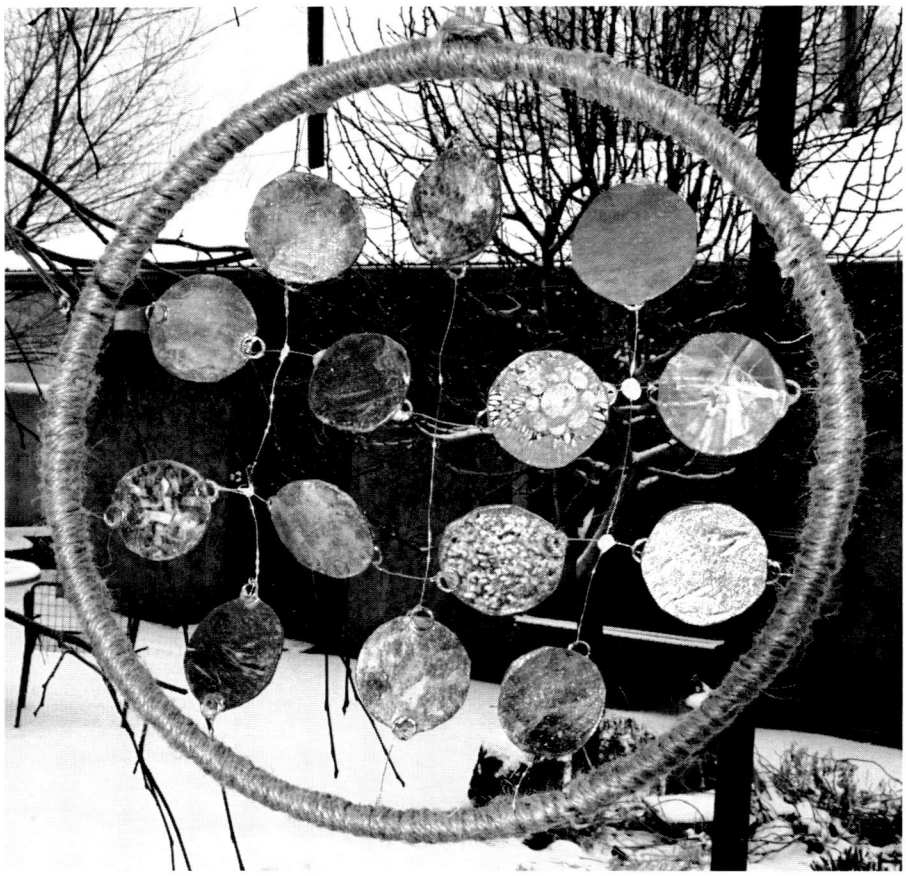

Figure 14. Connecting the Dots, Wendy Wasserman.

The rough edges speak to Wendy of the rough, uncomfortable places in family life and the circles are symbolic of her current work to "connect the dots" of her life. The little circles are a little "off" in Wendy's eyes and she felt strongly about not changing this art piece into something that it's not. The difficult family stories are still present in this genogram, nothing has been taken away or dismissed. Instead, something significant has been added. Wendy described how she took the circles and used her fingers, touching each circle gently with the shiny gold paint. Her art-based genogram has a subtle shimmer and it definitely catches the light. Wendy's words eloquently sum up what my heart hopes for as people grapple with the shadowy parts of family life. She has found a way to hold both, the sadness and now the hope, when she says "There is light in this family still."

REFERENCES

Badenoch, B. (2008). *Being a brain-wise therapist.* New York, NY: W. W. Norton & Company.

Berry, J. K. (2011). *Personal geographies; Explorations in mixed-media mapmaking.* Cinncinati, OH: Northern Lights Books.

Bowen, M. (1978). *Family therapy in clinical practice.* Northvale, NJ: Jason Aronson.

Bradshaw, J. (1988). *Healing the shame that binds you.* Deerfield Beach, FL: Health Communications.

Bradshaw, J. (1995). *Family secrets: The path from shame to healing.* New York, NY: Bantam Books.

Brooke, S. L. (2004). *Tools of the trade: A therapist's guide to art therapy assessments* (2nd ed.). Springfield, IL: Charles C Thomas.

Cozolino, L. (2006). *The neuroscience of human relationships, attachment and the developing social brain.* New York, NY: W. W. Norton & Company.

Dias, B. G., & Ressler, K. J. (2013). Parental olfactory experience influences behavior and neural structure in subsequent generations. *Nature Neuroscience,* Vol:17 (1), 89–96. doi: 10.1038/nn.3594.

Fein, J. (2014). *The spoon from minkowitz: A bittersweet roots journey to ancestral lands.* Santa Fe, NM: A GlobalAdventure.us book.

Fossum, M. A., & Mason, M. J. (1986). *Facing shame: Families in recovery.* New York, NY: W. W. Norton & Company.

Gibson, R. (2008). *My body, my earth: The practice of somatic archeology.* Bloomington, IN: iUniverse.

Gil, E. (1994). *Play in family therapy.* New York, NY: Guilford Press.

Gottman, J. M., & Silver, N. (1999). *The seven principles for making marriage work.* New York, NY: Crown Publishers Inc.

Haines, S. (2007). *Healing sex: A mind-body approach to healing sexual trauma.* San Francisco, CA: Cleis Press Inc.

Hautman Bates, A. (2014). *Mapping out family systems with genogram oil painting.* http://swc.edu/blogs/top-news/mapping-out-family-systems-with-genogram-oil-painting/#.U9FIC2dU.

Higgins-Klein, D. (2013). *Mindfulness-based play-family therapy: Theory and practice.* New York, NY: W. W. Norton & Company.

Hinz, L. D. (2006). *Drawing from within: Using art to treat eating disorders.* London, England: Jessica Kingsley.

Johnston, A. (1996). *Eating in the light of the moon.* Carlsbad, CA: Gurze Books.

Kerr, M. E., & Bowen, M. (1988). *Family evaluation: An approach based on Bowen theory.* New York, NY: W. W. Norton & Company.

Kerr, C., Hoshino, J., Sutherland, J., Thode Parashak, S., & McMarley, L. L. (2008). *Family art therapy: Foundations of theory and practice.* New York, NY: Routledge.

Kronberg, R., & McKissack, P. C. (1990). *A piece of the wind: And other stories to tell.* New York, NY: Harper & Row.

Kwiatkowska, H. Y. (1978). *Family therapy and evaluation through art.* Springfield, IL: Charles C Thomas.

Landgarten, H. B. (1987). *Family art psychotherapy: A clinical guide and casebook.* New York, NY: Brunner/Mazel.

Lerner, H. G. (1985). *The dance of anger: A woman's guide to changing the patterns of intimate relationships.* New York, NY: Harper & Row.

Linesch, D. (2000). *Celebrating family milestones by making art together.* Buffalo, NY: Firefly books.

Malchiodi, C. A., & Steele, W. (2008). Interventions for parents of traumatized children. In C. A. Malchiodi (Ed.), *Creative interventions with traumatized children.* New York, NY: Guilford Press.

Malchiodi, C. A. (2012). *Handbook of art therapy.* (2nd ed.). New York, NY: Guilford Press.

Maté, G. (2009). *In the realm of Hungry ghosts: Close encounters with addiction.* Berkeley, CA: North Atlantic Books.

McGoldrick, M., Gerson, R., & Petry, S. (2008). *Genograms: Assessment and intervention* (3rd ed.). New York, NY: W. W. Norton & Company.

McGoldrick, M. (2011). *The genogram journey: Reconnecting with your family.* New York, NY: W. W. Norton & Company.

McNiff, S. (1992). *Art as medicine: Creating a therapy of the imagination.* Boston MA: Shambhala.

Moon, C. H. (2010). *Materials & media in art therapy: Critical understandings of diverse artistic vocabularies.* New York, NY: Routledge.

Pipher, M. (1996). *The shelter of each other: Rebuilding our families.* New York, NY: G. P. Putnam's Sons.

Richards, P. S., Hardman, R. K., & Berrett, M. E. (2007). *Spiritual approaches in the treatment of women with eating disorders.* Washington, D.C.: American Psychological Association.

Riley, S. (2004). *Family art therapy* (2nd ed.). Chicago, IL: Magnolia Street Publishers.

Satir, V. (1983). *Conjoint family therapy* (3rd ed.). Palo Alto, CA: Science and Behavior Books.

Satir, V. (1972). *Peoplemaking.* Palo Alto, CA: Science and Behavior Books.

Schaeffer, C. (2006). *Grandmothers counsel the world: Women elders offer their vision for our planet.* Boston, MA: Trumpeter.

Schwartz, R. C. (2001). *Introduction to the internal family systems model.* Oak Park, IL: Trailhead Publications.

Siegel, D. J. (1999). *The developing mind: How relationships and the brain interact to shape who we are.* New York, NY: Guilford Press.

Singh, A. A., & Harper, A. (2012). Intercultural issues in LGBTQQ couple and family therapy. In J. J. Bigner & J. L. Wetchler (Eds.), *Handbook of lbgt-affirmative couple and family therapy.* New York, NY: Routledge.

Soll, J. (2000). *Adoption healing . . . a path to recovery.* Baltimore, MD: Gateway Press.

Solomon, A. (2012). *Far from the tree: Parents, children and the search for identity.* New York, NY: Scribner.

Weeks, G. R., & Fife, S. T. (2014) *Couples in treatment: Techniques and approaches for effective practice* (3rd ed.). New York, NY: Routledge.

Weiser, J. (1999). *PhotoTherapy techniques: Exploring the secrets of personal snapshots and family albums.* Vancouver, BC: PhotoTherapy Centre.

INDEX

A

addiction. *see* substance abuse
Allena, Thom, 29–30
arguments, 44–45
art therapy. *see also* therapy
    assessment, 34
    creating genograms, 17–24
    directive/nondirective, 55
    purpose, v, vii
    teaching, 5–6, 17
    temporary, 23–24
    use of, 11–16

B

Bowen, Murray, 4–5

C

childrens therapy. *see* therapy
collaboration, 99–104
counseling, marriage, 46. *see also* therapy, couples
couples therapy. *see* therapy
creating, 17–24

D

disabilities, physical, 37–38
Doggie genogram, 55–62

E

eating disorders, 88–92
"emotional genealogy," 26–27. *see also* generations
employment issues, 87–88
ethnicity. *see* multicultural issues

F

Family Puppet Interviews, 58–59
family systems theory
    family portraits (abstract), 13
    origin of, 4–5
    principles, 7
family therapy. *see* therapy
Feelings genogram, 45

G

generations (family)
    ancestry, 14–15, 25–28
        family history meetings, 59
        family stories, 49
    "emotional genealogy," 26–27
    reaching adulthood, 7
    relationships, ix, 6
    somatic archeology, 28
    special issues, 87–94
genograms
    and couples therapy, 41–47
    creating, 14
    defined, 4–6
    deviations from traditional, 11–12
    Doggie, 55–62
    and family therapy, 49–54
    Feelings, 45
    and generations (family)
        family map, 60–61
        special issues, 87–94
    history of, 3–10
    and individual therapy, 33–39

metaphors
  ancestry, 28–29
  animals, 15–16, 50, 55–56, 61, 64
  beds, 42
  candles, 50
  cards, 35–36
  chess, 21
  food/dessert, 20–21, 34–35, 73–75
  gardens, 63–67
  glaciers, 69–72
  gold, 65
  landscapes, 15
  materials, chosen, 21–23
  traumatic, 51–52, 74–75
  volcanoes, 3–4
  weather, 39
  and multicultural issues, 77–85
  and quilting, 20
  and repressed issues, 95–98
  revisions, 105–110
  standard, 11, 18
  teaching, 17, 19
  as temporary art, 23–24
Gibson, Rudy, 28

H

health issues
  crisis, 53
  insurance/affordability, 26
history of, 3–10
  value in family therapy, 25–32

I

identity, horizontal, 37–38
individual therapy. *see* therapy
inner community, 100–101
intimacy, 41–42. *see also* therapy, couples

K

Kwiatkowska, Hannah Yaxa, 13

L

Landgarten, Helen, 52

M

metaphors
  ancestry, 28–29
  animals
    birds, 64
    dogs, 55–56
    dolphins, 50
    elk, 15–16
    foxes, 61
    jellyfish, 15–16
  beds, 42
  candles, 50
  food/dessert, 20–21, 34–35, 73–75
    eating disorders, 88–92
  games
    cards, 35–36
    chess, 21
  geographic
    gardens, 63–67
    glaciers, 69–72
    landscapes, 15, 30
    volcanoes, 3–4
  gold, 65
  materials, chosen, 21–23
    natural, 107–108
    printed materials, 37, 65
    sculpture, 58, 81, 111–112
    textiles, 83–84
  mortality, 9
  traumatic, 51–52, 74–75
  weather, 39
multicultural issues, 77–85

P

portraits, family (abstract), 13

Q

quilting, 20

R

repressed issues, 95–98
"restorative circles," 29
revisions, 105–110
rituals and ceremonies, 30–31

Index

S

Satir, Virginia, 6, 58, 62
"self-geography map," 79
sexual identity
    LGBTQQ, 47
    parent's jealousy, 90
somatic archeology, 28. *see also* generations
substance abuse, 92–93
symbols, 13–14. *see also* metaphors

T

"terra psychology," 30
therapy. *see also* art therapy
    childrens. *see also* therapy, family
        introducing, 55–62
        uses of genograms, 55–62
    couples
        marriage, 46, 77–78
        uses of genograms, 41–47
    family. *see also* therapy, childrens
        crisis, 53
        history, value of, 25–32
        "restorative circles," 29
        uses of genograms, 49–54
    individual
        "self-geography map," 79
        uses of genograms, 33–39

CHARLES C THOMAS • PUBLISHER, LTD.

BECOMING AN ART THERAPIST
By Maxine Borowsky Junge & Kim Newall
2015, 184 pp. (7 x 10), 13 il.
$34.95 (paper), $34.95 (ebook)

THERAPISTS CREATING A CULTURAL TAPESTRY
By Stephanie L. Brooke & Charles E. Myers
2015, 344 pp. (7 x 10), 21 il.
$62.95 (hard), $62.95 (ebook)

ATTUNEMENT IN EXPRESSIVE ARTS THERAPY
By Mitchell Kossak
2015, 184 pp. (7 x 10), 25 il.
$28.95 (paper), $28.95 (ebook)

THE USE OF CREATIVE THERAPIES IN TREATING DEPRESSION
By Stephanie L. Brooke & Charles E. Myers
2015, 368 pp. (7 x 10), 38 il.
$69.95 (hard), $69.95 (ebook)

THE ART THERAPISTS' PRIMER (2nd Ed.)
By Ellen G. Horovitz
2014, 380 pp. (7 x 10), 102 il., 2 tables.
$74.95 (hard), $74.95 (ebook)

ART-BASED GROUP THERAPY
By Bruce L. Moon
2010, 180 pp. (7 x 10), 18 il.
$34.95 (paper), $34.95 (ebook)

ART, ANGST, AND TRAUMA
By Doris Banowsky Arrington
2007, 278 pp. (7 x 10), 123 il.
$48.95 (paper), $48.95 (ebook)

TOOLS OF THE TRADE (2nd Ed.)
By Stephanie L. Brooke
2004, 256 pp. (7 x 10), 19 il.
$59.95 (hard), $39.95 (paper), $39.95 (ebook)

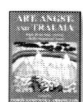
THE ART AND SCIENCE OF EVALUATION IN THE ARTS THERAPIES (2nd Ed.)
By Robyn Flaum Cruz & Bernard Feder
2013, 420 pp. (7 x 10), 11 il., 5 tables.
$73.95 (hard), $53.95 (paper), $53.95 (ebook)

SPIRITUAL ART THERAPY (2nd Ed.)
By Ellen G. Horovitz
2002, 220 pp. (7 x 10), 47 il., 2 tables.
$37.95 (paper), $37.95 (ebook)

THE MODERN HISTORY OF ART THERAPY IN THE UNITED STATES
By Maxine Borowsky Junge
2010, 370 pp. (7 x 10), 19 il., 1 table.
$77.95 (hard), $57.95 (paper), $57.95 (ebook)

THEY COULD NOT TALK AND SO THEY DREW
By Myra F. Levick
1983, 240 pp., 134 il., 11 tables.
$52.95 (paper), $52.95 (ebook)

ART THERAPY WITH OLDER ADULTS
By Rebecca C. Perry Magniant
2004, 256 pp. (7 x 10), 26 il., 2 tables.
$39.95 (paper), $39.95 (ebook)

INTEGRATING THE ARTS IN THERAPY
By Shaun McNiff
2009, 280 pp. (7 x 10), 60 il.
$59.95 (hard), $39.95 (paper), $39.95 (ebook)

ART FOR ALL THE CHILDREN (2nd Ed.)
By Frances E. Anderson
1992, 398 pp. (6.75 x 9.75), 113 il., 19 tables.
$62.95 (paper), $62.95 (ebook)

ETHICAL ISSUES IN ART THERAPY (2nd Ed.)
By Bruce L. Moon
2006, 290 pp. (7 x 10), 21 il.
$59.95 (hard), $59.95 (ebook)

IDENTITY AND ART THERAPY
By Maxine Borowsky Junge
2014, 250 pp. (7 x 10)
$39.95 (paper), $39.95 (ebook)

ART THERAPY WITH STUDENTS AT RISK (2nd Ed.)
By Stella A. Stepney
2009, 222 pp. (7 x 10), 16 il., 19 tables.
$59.95 (hard), $39.95 (paper), $39.95 (ebook)

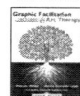
GRAPHIC FACILITATION AND ART THERAPY
By Michelle Winkel & Maxine Borowsky Junge
2012, 178 pp. (7 x 10), 14 il.
$35.95 (paper), $35.95 (ebook)

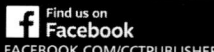
Find us on Facebook
FACEBOOK.COM/CCTPUBLISHER

TO ORDER: 1-800-258-8980 • books@ccthomas.com • www.ccthomas.com